# Fast and Flavorful Paleo Cooking [3 Books in 1]

## The Ultimate Cookbook with 150+ Te͏                     ͏d Kid-Friendly Recipes for Everyday

**Chef John Tank**

# Author : Chef John Tank

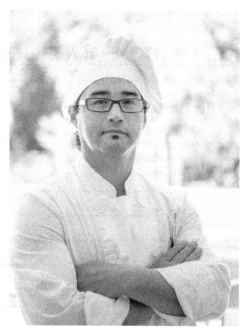

Chef John Tank is the leading authority on the science and application of the carnivore diet. He used his best years of experience to build the perfect diet recipes to reverse self-immunity, chronic inflammation and mental health problems helping hundreds of people. Chef John Tank went viral after showing some of his best recipes through social networks in the late 2018. The great reviews spurred him to find the perfect medium to teach him about his delicious masterpieces. Here we can officially celebrate the 7 new releases of Chef John Tank taken from the brand-new series: "The Butcher Boot Camp". A real collection of kitchen manuals that will leave a mark on the palate of all your friends and family.

# Table of Contents

## PALEO DIET COOKBOOK

# THE 5-INGREDIENT PALEO DIET COOKBOOK

# QUICK PREP PALEO

# Paleo Diet Cookbook

*Manage Your Appetite and Kill Hunger Tasting. Tens of Easy and Healthy Recipes. Raise Body Energy, Balance Blood Glucose Levels, and Stay Paleo*

**By**

## Chef John Tank

# Contents

# Introduction

The Paleo diet, also known as the Stone-Age or caveman diet, contains nuts, lean meats, fruits, fish, vegetables, and seeds. Proponents of the diet emphasize preferring low-glycemic vegetables and fruit.

Paleo diet is high in protein, mild in fat (primarily from unsaturated fats), high in fiber, moderate-low in carbohydrate (specifically limiting the high glycemic index carbohydrates), and low in refined and sodium sugars. The polyunsaturated and monounsaturated fats (this includes the omega-3 fats DHA and EPA) come from avocado, marine fish, olive oil, seeds, and nuts.

Grass-fed beef is also emphasized on the paleo diet and is publicized to have more omega-3 fats than standard beef because of being fed grass rather than grain. It has minimal alpha-linolenic acid concentrations (ALA), which is a precursor to DHA and EPA. However, only a limited ALA proportion can be transformed in the organism to long-chain omega-3 fatty acids. The level of omega-3 is also extremely variable depending on the specific feeding routine and variations in fat metabolism across cattle breeds. Also, the level of omega-3 in grass-fed beef is much smaller than that in oily sea fish. Cooked salmon produces 1000-2000 mg of DHA/EPA per 3-ounce part, while 3 ounces of grass-fed beef contains between 20-200 mg of ALA.

While it is difficult to tell precisely what human predecessors consumed in various parts of the world, researchers suggest their diets consisted of whole foods.

By adopting a whole-food diet and maintaining active lives physically, hunter-gatherers likely had significantly lower rates of health risks and disorders, such as diabetes, obesity, and cardiac disease.

# Chapter 1: Introduction to Paleo Diet

The paleo diet is planned to reflect what human hunter-gatherer predecessors consumed in ancient times.

Many reports show that this diet will contribute to substantial weight loss but without counting calories and also lead to major improvements in health.

This section is a basic guide to the paleo diet, including a clear meal plan and other important details.

There is controversy on many aspects of the Paleo diet: what items existed at the time, the difference in diets based on the area (e.g., the Arctic vs. tropical), how modern-day vegetables and fruit show no similarity to ancient wild versions, and dispute among Paleo diet enthusiasts about what is excluded or included from the diet. Because of these variations, there is not one "true" Paleo diet.

For example, while white potatoes were documented to be present during the Paleolithic period, they are typically avoided in this diet due to their high glycemic mark. Processed foods are still off-limits technically due to a focus on fresh foods, but certain Paleo diets include frozen fruits and vegetables since the freezing process retains most nutrients.

## 1.1 A Paleo Diet Meal Plan

There is not a "right" way to adopt paleo. The paleolithic humans thrived on several diets based on what was accessible at the moment and where in the world they lived.

Some consumed a low-carb diet rich in animal foods, and others adopted a high-carb diet of plenty of plants.

Consider this as a basic guideline, not anything cast in concrete. It would be best if you customize all of this to your unique desires and interests.

Here are the basics:

**Eat:** Meat, eggs, fish, healthy fats, vegetables, nuts, fruits, seeds, spices, herbs, and oils.

**Avoid:** Soft drinks, processed foods, sugar, vegetable oils, grains, legumes, most dairy products, margarine, artificial sweeteners, and trans fats.

## 1.2 Foods to Eat on the Paleo Diet

Establish your diet on unprocessed and whole paleo foods:

- **Meat:** Beef, chicken, lamb, pork, turkey, and others.

- **Eggs:** Get pastured, omega-3 enriched or free-range eggs.

- **Healthy fats and oils:** coconut oil, Extra virgin olive oil, avocado oil, and others.

- **Vegetables:** Broccoli, peppers, kale, onions, tomatoes, carrots etc.

- **Fish and seafood:** Salmon, shellfish, haddock, trout, shrimp, etc. If you are able, choose wild-caught.

- **Fruits:** Apples, oranges, bananas, pears, strawberries, avocados, blueberries and more.

- **Nuts and seeds:** Almonds, walnuts, macadamia nuts, hazelnuts, pumpkin seeds, sunflower seeds and more.

- **Tubers:** Potatoes, sweet potatoes, yams, turnips, etc.

- **Salt and spices:** Sea salt, turmeric, garlic, rosemary, etc.

If you can afford it, consider preferring pasture-raised, grass-fed, and organic. In short, eat unprocessed, whole foods such as meat, seafood, eggs, fruits, veggies, potatoes, healthy fats, nuts, and spices. If not, then be sure you always reach with the least-processed alternative. Choose organic and grass-fed products where possible.

## 1.3 Foods to Avoid on the Paleo Diet

Avoid the following ingredients and food items:

- **High-fructose and sugar corn syrup:** Soft drinks, table sugar, fruit juices, candy, ice cream, pastries, and many others.

- **Grains:** Breads, rye, wheat, pastas, spelt, barley, etc.

- **Legumes:** Lentils, beans and many more.

- **Dairy:** Avoid dairy, especially the ones with low-fat (there are also some versions of paleo that include full-fat dairy like cheese and butter).

- **Some vegetable oils:** Soybean oil, grapeseed oil, cottonseed oil, sunflower oil, corn oil, safflower oil and others.

- **Trans fats:** Found in various processed foods and margarine. Usually called "partially hydrogenated" or "hydrogenated" oils.

- **Artificial sweeteners:** Aspartame, acesulfame potassium, cyclamates, sucralose, saccharin. You can use natural sweeteners instead.

- **Highly processed foods:** Products labeled "low-fat" or "diet" or that has many additives. These include artificial meal replacements.

A basic guideline: Do not consume it if it seems like it was manufactured in a factory.

You must review ingredient lists if you want to avoid certain additives, including items advertised as "healthy foods." In short, avoid all refined ingredients or foods, including bread, sugar, some trans fats, vegetable oils, and artificial sweeteners.

## 1.4 What to Drink When You are Thirsty

Water can be the go-to drink when it comes to hydration. The following beverages are not exactly paleo, but they are drunk by most people anyway:

- **Tea:** Tea is safe and filled with different antioxidants and beneficial compounds. The best is green tea.

- **Coffee:** Coffee is often very rich in antioxidants. Studies say that there are multiple health advantages of it.

## 1.5 Simple Paleo Snacks

There is no reason to consume more than three meals a day, but if you are starving, here are some quick and easy-to-carry paleo snacks:

- Hard-boiled eggs

- Baby carrots

- A handful of nuts

- A piece of fruit

- Apple with almond butter

- Leftovers from the last day

- Homemade beef jerky

- Berries with coconut cream

## 1.6 Sensible Indulgences

In limited quantities, the foods and drinks below are completely fine:

- **Wine:** Quality red wine is rich in antioxidants and nutrients that are helpful.

- **Dark chocolate:** Get the one that has a cocoa content of 70 percent or greater. The quality of dark chocolate is very healthy and very nutritional.

## 1.7 A Sample Paleo Menu for One Week

A healthy number of paleo-friendly foods is included in this sample menu.

Customize this menu depending on your preferences, by all means.

**Monday**

- **Breakfast:** Fried vegetables and eggs in coconut oil. Besides that, get a piece of fruit too.

- **Lunch:** Chicken salad along with olive oil. Besides that, some nuts.

- **Dinner:** Burgers (without bun) cooked in butter, with some salsa and vegetables.

**Tuesday**

- **Breakfast:** Eggs and bacon, with one piece of any fruit.

- **Lunch:** Burgers from the last night.

- **Dinner:** Salmon and with vegetables fried in butter.

**Wednesday**

- **Breakfast:** Vegetables and meat (leftovers from last night).

- **Lunch:** Sandwich with fresh vegetables and meat.

- **Dinner:** Stir fry ground beef with vegetables. Get some berries too.

## Thursday

- **Breakfast:** One piece of fruit and eggs.

- **Lunch:** Stir-fry. A handful of nuts.

- **Dinner:** Vegetables and fried pork.

## Friday

- **Breakfast:** Vegetables and eggs fried in coconut oil.

- **Lunch:** Chicken salad along with olive oil. Also eat some nuts.

- **Dinner:** Vegetables and steak. And some sweet potatoes.

## Saturday

- **Breakfast:** Eggs and bacon with a piece of fruit.

- **Lunch:** Steak and vegetables.

- **Dinner:** Baked salmon with avocado and vegetables.

## Sunday

- **Breakfast:** Meat along with vegetables.

- **Lunch:** Sandwich with fresh vegetables and meat.

- **Dinner:** Grilled chicken wings with salsa and vegetables.

Typically, there is no need to track macronutrients or calories (carbohydrates, protein, or fat) in the paleo diet, at least not at the beginning. However, if you want to lose a lot of weight, cutting carbohydrates more and restricting the consumption of high-fat items, such as nuts, is a smart option.

## 1.8 Simple Paleo Shopping List

On the paleo diet, there is an incredible number of things you may consume. You will get an overview of how to get started with this easy shopping list:

- **Meat:** Beef, pork, lamb, etc.

- **Poultry:** Turkey, chicken, etc.

- **Fish:** Salmon, mackerel, trout, etc.

- **Eggs**

- **Fresh vegetables:** Greens, tomatoes, lettuce, peppers, onions, carrots, etc.

- **Frozen vegetables:** Broccoli, various vegetable mixes, spinach, etc.

- **Fruits:** Apples, avocado, pears, bananas, oranges etc.

- **Berries:** Blueberries, strawberries, etc.

- **Nuts:** Almonds, macadamia nuts, walnuts, hazelnuts

- **Almond butter**

- **Coconut oil**

- **Olive oil**

- **Olives**

- **Sweet potatoes**

- **Condiments:** Sea salt, turmeric, parsley, pepper, garlic, etc.

Clearing all unhealthy cravings from your house, including ice cream, pastries, sugary sodas, cookies, bread, crackers, and cereals, is a smart idea. Next, fill your pantry and freezer with tasty, paleo-friendly ingredients and use the grocery list above.

## 1.9 Modified Paleo Diets

The paleo movement has grown quite a bit over the last few years.

Several separate variations of the paleo diet currently exist. Many of them cause certain modern foods to be safe, as evidence indicates.

These include quality butter that is fed with grass. There are also some grains for example, gluten-free rice.

Many people now think about paleo as a pattern, not just a rigid collection of guidelines that you have to obey to focus your diet on. You may still consider the paleo diet as a starting point, incorporating gluten-free grains and grass-fed butter alongside a few other balanced foods.

## 1.10 How to Make Restaurant Meals Paleo

Making the majority of restaurant meals paleo-friendly is pretty simple.

Some basic instructions are here:

1. Pick a main dish focused on meat-or fish.

2. Instead of rice or bread, get extra veggies.

3. Ask them to cook in coconut oil or olive oil for your meal.

Eating out does not have to be challenging when adopting the paleo diet. On the menu, easily pick a meat or fish dish and mix in some additional vegetables.

## 1.11 Pros

There are a handful of advantages from adopting the paleo diet that you might potentially enjoy.

Next, you will get all of the important vitamins and minerals you need through consuming fruits and vegetables.

The food is easy as well. There is no prepackaged meal schedule or diet loop to commit to, and you consume the suitable items and skip those that are not.

There are lots of benefits to it. Through juice or soft drinks, it takes out many processed foods only naturally, such as added sugar or processed grains. And since the diet encourages the intake of anti-inflammatory foods, such as vegetables, fruits, and unsaturated fats in certain oils and nuts, your wellbeing will benefit. Eating out refined foods and sweets would also reduce the chances of illnesses, such as type 2 diabetes and some cancers.

The diet, besides, emphasizes workout. Exercise is an integral part of a balanced lifestyle that will help you lose weight or maintain it.

## 1.12 Cons

A diet for hunter-gatherers can be hard to sustain, particularly in the long term. Since most foods are consumed

plain, within a short period, adopting the eating strategy may become tedious.

Foods that are organically raised may often be pricey, and grass-fed beef and other meats usually cost more.

For example, one model focused on data sets from the U.S. Department of Agriculture showed that it would be necessary to raise sales by 9 percent to adopt the paleo diet when fulfilling all recommended regular micronutrient inputs (except calcium).

And again, there is no concrete empirical evidence that the paleo diet avoids sickness. Any confirmation of its advantages is anecdotal. While the advantages of the paleo diet seem to be confirmed by several trials, many experts also claim that we do not yet have enough data to know if the dietary strategy is safe and risk-free. Nobody understands this diet's long-term consequences, and no one has studied it to some degree. It is not exactly a new concept; instead, it is something that has been repeated through the years.

The diet's fat allowance, for example, could be troublesome. As a better alternative, you might aim for locally sourced meat, whose sources and system of raising you are conscious of. An elevated probability of early death has been correlated with saturated fat from meat.

One research referenced in the paper, reported in the European Journal of Clinical Nutrition, showed that calcium consumption levels were as poor as 50 percent of the recommended daily value for paleo diet followers.

Calcium deficiency can induce symptoms such as tingling in the fingers, numbness and muscle cramps, lethargy (or loss of energy), convulsions, poor appetite, and irregular heart rhythms. Persistent calcium deficiency can result in skeletal disorders such as an increased risk of fractures, osteoporosis, and rickets.

A certified dietitian will help you implement this plan safely to prevent nutritional deficiencies such                                          as                                          calcium.

# Chapter 2: Health benefits of paleo

People say that multiple health advantages are offered by the paleo diet, including promoting weight reduction, lowering the risk of diabetes, and decreasing blood pressure.

In this section, we aim at the scientific evidence and see whether all of these claims are supported by research:

## 2.1 Weight loss

An earlier 2008 research showed that by adopting the paleo diet for three weeks, 14 fit participants obtained an overall weight loss of 2.3 kilograms.

Researchers contrasted the impact of a paleo diet with a diabetes diet on 13 persons with type 2 diabetes in 2009. The small research showed that eating the paleo diet reduced the body weight and waist circumference of participants.

A 2014 survey of 70 postmenopausal overweight women showed that participants helped reduce weight after six months on a paleo diet.

However, there was a little gap in weight reduction after two years for participants adopting the paleo diet as well as those adhering to standard guidelines for Nordic nutrition. Such studies indicate that some healthier diets could be almost as important in encouraging weight loss.

The writers of a 2017 study acknowledged that the paleo diet helps lose weight in the short term but argued that this effect is attributed to caloric limits or fewer calories eaten.

Overall, the study shows that the paleo diet can initially help individuals lose weight, but other diets that limit calorie consumption can be just as successful.

Before doctors prescribe the paleo diet for weight reduction, further study is required. Doctors currently encourage individuals to adopt a calorie-controlled diet and to work out more to reduce weight.

## 2.2 Reducing diabetes risk.

Can a person's chance of developing diabetes be lowered by adopting a paleo diet plan? The outcomes of some initial research are encouraging.

A risk factor for diabetes is insulin resistance. Improving the insulin sensitivity of an individual reduces the risk that they may have diabetes which will help their effects among people who have diabetes.

In 2015, a small review contrasted the paleo diet results with that of a diet focused on American Diabetes Association guidelines on persons with type 2 diabetes.

Although both diets increased the patients' metabolic well-being, enhancing insulin tolerance and blood sugar regulation was higher with the paleo diet.

Earlier research in 2009 of nine sedentary participants without obesity has shown that insulin regulation was increased by the paleo diet.

A more recent study on the paleo diet and diabetes is required, but the evidence to date shows that living like a hunter-gatherer can increase the sensitivity to insulin.

## 2.3 Lowering blood pressure.

A risk factor for cardiac failure is high blood pressure. Some individuals claim that the paleo diet will help regulate blood pressure and improve cardiac wellbeing.

Earlier research in 2008 of 14 active participants showed that systolic blood pressure improved during a paleo diet for three weeks. It also decreased weight and the index of body mass (BMI). However, the research did not involve a control group, so the conclusions are not conclusive.

These early results were followed by a 2014 report. The researchers contrasted the results of a paleo diet to a diet prescribed by the Dutch Health Council for 34 participants with metabolic syndrome characteristics, a disorder that raises the risk of cardiac disease.

Results found that blood lipid and blood pressure profiles were lowered by the paleo diet, which can promote cardiac health.

While initial studies indicate that the paleo diet can decrease blood pressure and improve cardiac health, more recent and detailed studies are required to draw some conclusions.

## 2.4 Is the Paleo Diet Good for Heart Health?

The paleo diet, as with type 2 diabetes, can or may not be healthy for your heart. It comes down to how you adopt the method to eating.

If you were to consume an unlimited amount of red meat (which is technically allowed by the paleo diet), you will most definitely develop cardiac health issues. Although experts applaud the exclusion of canned and refined items such as cake, chips, cookies, and candy, widely established to be bad for your ticker, they are not crazy that paleo would not encourage you to ingest whole legumes, grains, and most dairy goods. In fact, whole grains have been related to higher levels of cholesterol, as well as a decreased risk of obesity, stroke, and type 2 diabetes.

There are cardiac disorder co-morbidities.

Before attempting the paleo diet for heart disease, consult with the specialist. He or she would be able to inform you if that is a suitable match, and if not, if the optimal health strategy can be handled.

## 2.5 Is Paleo a Good Choice If You Have Diabetes?

While there is no ideal diet for diabetes, some evidence indicates that the emphasis of the paleo diet on whole foods can help individuals with type 2 diabetes lower their blood pressure, control their blood sugar, and lose weight.

Critics claim that in those with diabetes, the limitless amount of red meat that the paleo diet requires can have a detrimental impact on cardiac wellbeing, as evidence ties consuming red meat in abundance to impaired heart health.

This may be a major concern if you have diabetes and do not moderate the red-meat diet, since individuals with diabetes are twice as likely to suffer of heart failure as people without diabetes.

The takeaway: Ultimately, there are not sufficiently promising research findings for clinicians to make a specific decision to try the paleo diet for people with diabetes just yet. Make sure to clear up with the healthcare professional first if you intend to try the plan in order to control your blood sugar.

# Chapter 3: Breakfast Recipes

A balanced breakfast can be tough for just about everyone. The breakfast might seem much more overwhelming for anyone stuck to a Paleo diet.

For Paleo newcomers, eggs are still a choice, but going through several cartons a week gets old quickly. Besides, no one has to sacrifice the pancakes, waffles, and muffins.

Whenever you want nutrition-packed meals to begin your day, turn to the following paleo breakfast recipes.

## 1. Paleo Lemon Blueberry Bread

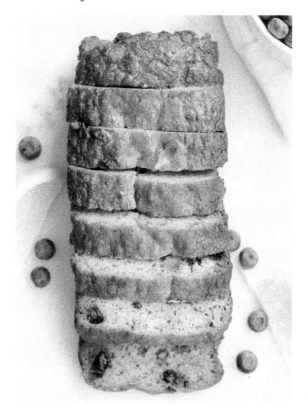

Prep time: 10 minutes

Cook time: 50 minutes

Total time: 1 hour

Servings: 1 bread

## Ingredients

- 2.5 tablespoons coconut flour

- 2 cups almond flour

- 1.5 teaspoon baking soda

- 2 tablespoons almond milk

- 3 eggs

- 1/4 cup maple syrup or honey

- 1/4 cup melted coconut oil.

- 2 smalls, mashed, very ripe bananas.

- 1 cup fresh blueberries

- Zest and juice of 1 lemon

## Instructions

1. Preheat the oven to 350°F.

2. In a medium dish, combine the coconut flour, almond flour, and baking soda.

3. Combine in a different bowl all the wet ingredients except the blueberries. Fill the dry ingredients with the wet ingredients and mix to combine. Fold in the blueberries gently.

4. 4.Line an 8x4 inch parchment paper in a loaf pan and pour your batter into it.

5. Bake for 25 minutes, then cover completely with foil and bake for 25-35 more minutes. The surface should be nicely browned, and a knife should come out clean placed in the middle.

6. Before cutting, remove from the pan and allow cool completely.

## 2. Stuffed Sweet Potato Burritos

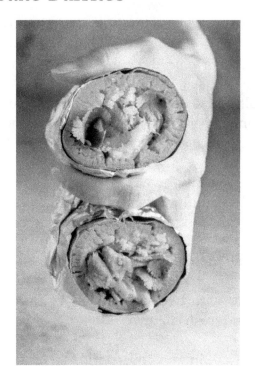

Prep Time: 2 minutes

Cook Time: 10 minutes

Total Time: 12 minutes

Servings: 1-2

## Ingredients

- 1/4 cup cauliflower rice

- 1 sweet potato

- juice of 1/2 small lime

- 1/2 teaspoon olive oil

- 1/3 cup cooked and shredded chicken.

- salt for taste

- 1 small handful of fresh cilantros

- 2 tablespoons salsa Verde

## Instructions

1. Wash the sweet potato, pat it off, and slice it with a sharp knife a few times.

2. Put for 6-8 minutes in the microwave until the inside is soft enough to scoop out.

3. Cut the sweet potato in half and scoop the inside out carefully, leaving a small amount of sweet potato along the skin's inner perimeter. If needed, save the remaining sweet potato mash for a different meal.

4. In a small saucepan, mix in the cauliflower rice and add the olive oil. Sauté for 3-4 minutes over medium-high heat until the cauliflower is soft. Over the cauliflower rice, squeeze the lime juice and combine. Add salt to taste and remove from the heat before ready to assemble.

5. Reheat and add the salsa Verde to the shredded chicken.   Mix well,

6. Layer each half of the burrito with two tablespoons of cauliflower rice, then sprinkle with shredded chicken salsa Verde and fresh cilantro.

7.     Serve     or     wrap     in     foil. (remove     the foil     if     microwaving)

## 3. Paleo Banana and Strawberry Cereal Bars

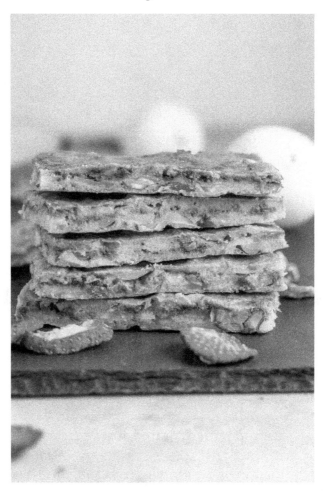

Prep Time: 10 minutes

Cook Time: 20 minutes

Total Time: 30 minutes

Servings: 12 bars

**Ingredients**

- 3 loaded tablespoons cashew butter

- 2 large ripe bananas

- 1/2 teaspoon vanilla extract

- 2 egg whites

- 1/2 cup finely sliced almonds

- 1 tablespoon coconut flour

- 1-ounce dehydrated strawberries

- 1/8 teaspoon salt

**Instructions**

1. Preheat your oven to 350 degrees F.

2. In a mini chopper or small food processor, put dehydrated strawberries and process them until they are broken down into crumbles.

3. 3.In a medium dish, add the cashew butter, egg whites, ripe bananas, and vanilla extract. Mix well,

4. 4. Add the flour and salt from the coconut and mix well to combine. Fold it  in the sliced almonds.

5. Grease a pan measuring 8-8". Split the batter in two,

6. Into the pan, add half the batter and distribute uniformly (it will spread thinly)

7. Sprinkle uniformly over the top of dehydrated strawberries.

8. Pour the left batter over the top of the strawberries that have been dehydrated.

9. Bake for 20 minutes before cutting into bars, then let it cool.

## 4. Paleo Porridge With Caramelized Bananas

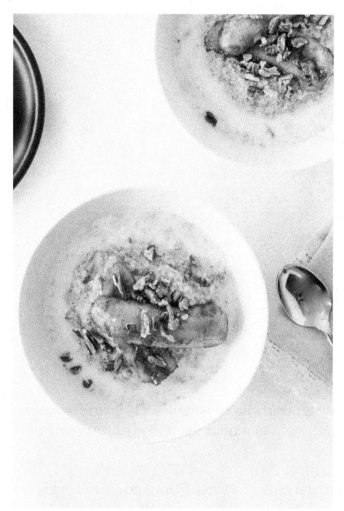

Prep Time: 10 mins

Cook Time: 20 mins

Total: 30 mins

Servings: 4 servings

**Ingredients**

- 1 cup raw cashews

- 1 cup raw pecans

- 4 pitted Medjool dates

- 2 cups coconut milk

- 1 tsp vanilla extract

- 1 tbsp chia seeds

- 1/4 tsp sea salt

## Caramelized Bananas

- 1 tbsp butter or ghee

- 2 bananas

- 1/4 tsp cinnamon

- 1 1/2 tbsp maple syrup

- 1 cup coconut milk

- 1/2 cup chopped pecans.

## Instructions

1. In a big bowl of water, put the nuts and soak them for 8 hours or overnight. Not only does soaking the nuts help to render the porridge smooth, but it also helps to improve the nuts' digestibility.

2. In a colander, drain the nuts and rinse them under the cool spray.

3. In a food processor, put the vanilla, nuts, chia, dates, and sea salt and process until finely ground.

4. To a pot, transfer the nut mixture. Add the coconut milk and turn the heat to medium-high. Remove from the heat and stir until hot and smooth.

5. Peel and split the bananas in two, and slice lengthwise again.

6. On medium heat, heat a skillet and add maple syrup, butter, and cinnamon, mixing until combined. Put the bananas and cook for one minute in the pan, then gently turn and cook on the other side for an additional minute.

7. Divide into four bowls of porridge. To each bowl, add a sprinkle of chopped pecans, caramelized bananas, and 1/4 cup of coconut milk.

## 5. Chunky Grain-Free Granola

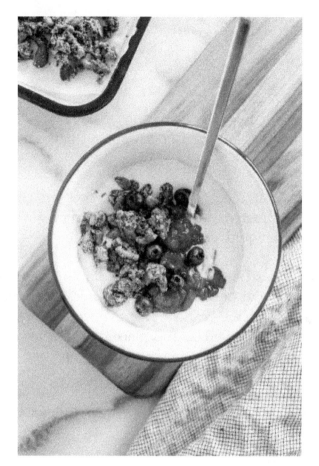

Prep time: 10 minutes

Cook time: 20 minutes.

Total time: 30 minutes

servings: 7

**Ingredients**

- 3/4 cup mixed seeds

- 2 cups chopped mixed nuts.

- 1/2 cup almond flour

- 1/2 cup unsweetened shredded coconut

- 1/2 teaspoon fine sea salt

- 1 teaspoon ground cinnamon

- 3 tablespoons pure maple syrup

- 3 tablespoons melted coconut oil.

- 1 teaspoon vanilla extract

## Instructions

1. Line a baking tray with a silicone mat or parchment paper and preheat the oven to 325 ° F.

2. Combine the almond flour, seeds, chopped nuts, coconut, cinnamon and salt in a large bowl. Pour the vanilla extract, melted coconut oil, and maple syrup over the top. Stir until it is covered equally with liquid.

3. On the baking sheet, spread the mixture out into a large rectangle. Transfer to the oven that has been preheated and bake for 20-25 minutes. The nuts will appear golden, and they should be fragrant with the granola. Remove from the oven and allow to cool totally before stirring. Transfer to a sealed jar and place for up to 1 week in the refrigerator.

## NOTES

The recipe yields about seven cups. The size of the serving equals 1/2 cup.

In place of maple syrup, you can add agave, honey, or coconut sugar. You may require adding a tablespoon of water or oil for moisture if you use coconut sugar.

# 6. Light Creamy Strawberry Chia Pudding

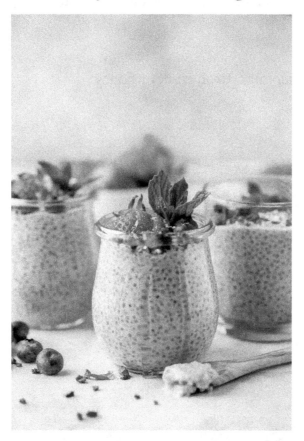

Cook Time: 3 hours 30 minutes

Total Time: 4 hours 5 minutes

Servings : 4

## Ingredients

- 1 can of full fat coconut milk (13.5 oz)

- 1 cup fresh strawberries

- 1 teaspoon vanilla bean paste

- 2 tablespoons raw honey

- 1/4 cup chia seeds

## Instructions

1. Add the honey, coconut milk, fresh strawberries and vanilla bean paste to a food processor or blender. Blend until you have pureed strawberries, and all is blended.

2. Add this mixture together with the chia seeds to a medium bowl. Mix all together with a spoon. Cover and leave for 4 hours or overnight to rest.

3. serve!

4. Optional: top with cacao nibs, fresh fruit, or honey

## 7. Sweet Potato Hash

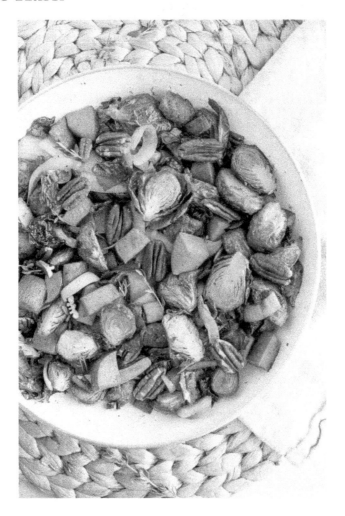

Prep Time: 10 minutes

Cook Time: 40 minutes

Total Time: 50 minutes

Servings: 3

**Ingredients**

- 1 lb. quartered brussels sprouts

- 1 medium sweet potato chopped finely into bite-size chunks.

- 1 1/2 Tablespoons and 2 teaspoons olive oil or avocado oil

- 3 frozen links of turkey, veggie, or chicken breakfast sausage

- 1/2 teaspoon sea salt and some more for taste

- 1/4 teaspoon paprika

- 1 chopped yellow onion.

- 1/4 teaspoon ground pepper and some more for taste

- 2 cups baby spinach

- 1 clove garlic

- 1/2 Tablespoon maple syrup (optional)

- 1 Tablespoon balsamic vinegar

- 3 poached or fried eggs

- 1/3 cup roughly chopped pecans

- fresh thyme, for serving.

- hot sauce, for serving.

## Instructions

1. Preheat the oven to 425 degrees F.

2. Add 1 1/2 tablespoons of oil,1/4 teaspoon paprika, 1/2 teaspoon salt, and 1/4 teaspoon pepper to the brussels sprouts and chopped sweet potatoes.

3. Spread the vegetables on a large baking sheet for 30-40 minutes and roast. Take the pan from the oven at the 25-minute mark, toss the vegetables and add the frozen sausage links to the sheet pan. Continue roasting until fork tender is sweet potatoes and sprouts, and sausage is warm throughout.

4. Meanwhile, toast the pecans for 1 to 2 minutes in a wide, dry skillet until they are golden brown. Watch carefully because they can rapidly burn. Remove from the heat, leave to cool, and then chop roughly.

5. Add two teaspoons of oil over medium-high flame, utilizing the same large skillet. Add the onions and garlic once the oil is hot. Season with a little pepper and sea salt and toss to mix. Cook for around 5-6 minutes until the onions are translucent and fragrant. To mix, add balsamic vinegar, baby spinach, and maple syrup and toss. Cook for around 1-2 minutes or until the spinach wilts. Remove from the heat and cover to keep warm until the vegetables are done roasting.

6. After roasting the brussels sprouts, sweet potatoes, and sausage, move them with the spinach and onion mixture to the skillet, add the pecans and toss it to combine, using the spatula to break the sausage links into smaller parts. To serve over the hash, cover to stay warm as you cook your eggs. However, you like, you may pan-fry or poach the eggs.

7. Place the sweet potato hash mixture on a plate and line it with two cooked eggs to serve. Garnish with fresh thyme and top with hot sauce.

NOTE

You should cook the roasted vegetables and the spinach and onion mixture 1-2 days in advance to save time. When you are about to serve, reheat on the stovetop when cooking your eggs.

## 8. Peanut Butter Oatmeal

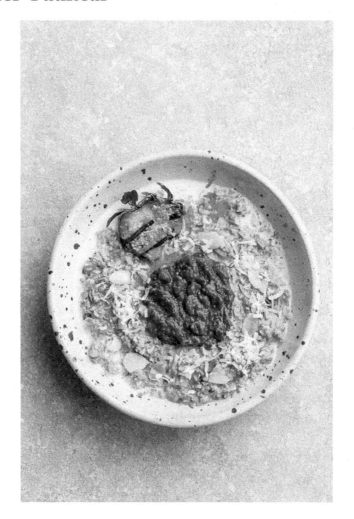

Prep Time: 5 mins

Cook Time: 5 mins

Total Time: 10 mins

Servings: 2

**Ingredients**

- 1/4 cup hemp seeds

- 1/2 cup flaked unsweetened coconut.

- 1/2 cup water

- 1 tablespoon coconut flour

- 1 tablespoon unsalted and drippy peanut butter, you can also use 1 1/2 teaspoons of sugar free and pure peanut powder.

- 1/3 cup canned coconut milk (full fat)

## TOPPINGS: (optional)

- Homemade Strawberry Chia Jam

- hemp seeds

- sliced almonds

- almond butter

- unsweetened shredded coconut

## Instructions

1. Using a medium saucepan to add coconut flour, hemp seeds, coconut, water & milk.

2. Carry it to a boil, then cook until thickened for 2 minutes. Add peanut powder or peanut butter, vanilla and cinnamon until combined.

3. Serve with optional toppings and more milk.

## 9. Banana Bread Waffles

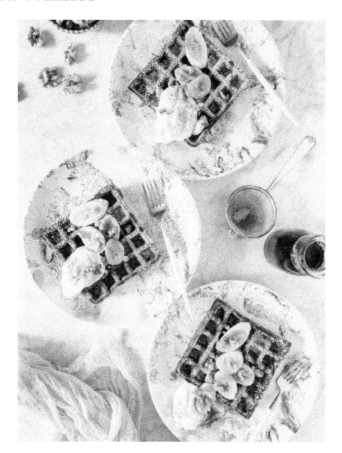

Prep time: 20 minutes

Cook time: 10 minutes

Total Time: 30 minutes

Servings: 6 large Belgian-style waffles

**Ingredients**

For the Bread Banana Waffles

- 1/3 cup melted coconut oil (2.65 ounces)

- 1/2 cup maple syrup (5.5 ounces)

- 2 large eggs, at room temperature

- 1/4 cup coconut milk (2 ounces)

- 1 3/4 cups Bob's Red Mill Paleo Baking Flour (7 ounces)

- 1 cup super ripe bananas (8 ounces)

- 1 teaspoon ground cinnamon

- 1 teaspoon Baking Soda

- 1/2 teaspoon kosher salt

For Serving

- fresh sliced bananas

- coconut whipped cream or coconut yogurt.

- maple syrup

- coarsely chopped walnuts

**Instructions**

1. Place a sheet pan in the center of the oven rack and preheat to 200 degrees F. According to the manufacturer's directions, preheat your waffle maker.

2. Whisk 1/3 cup of melted coconut oil, 1/2 cup of maple syrup, and 1/4 cup of coconut milk into a large bowl. Add two large eggs and whisk well. Add 1 cup of super ripe bananas and mix them into a thick puree using a stiff spatula or wooden spoon and spread the bananas over the batter.

3. Toss one teaspoon of ground cinnamon, one teaspoon of Baking Soda, 1 3/4 cups of Paleo Baking Flour, and 1/2 teaspoon of kosher salt together in a medium dish. Over the wet batter mixture, sprinkle the dry ingredients and use a wooden spoon to combine.

4. In the preheated waffle maker, cook the waffles using the proper amount of batter and the manufacturer's suggested time until golden. Shift to the preheated oven when the waffles finish cooking to keep them warm until the rest of the batter is done cooking; put each waffle directly on the middle rack of the oven. Serve immediately with chopped walnuts, freshly sliced bananas, and maple syrup with a coconut whipped cream or dollop of coconut yogurt. Enjoy!

# Chapter 4: Lunch Recipes

It can be challenging for everyone to escape from their workplace to get lunch, but lunchtime can be much more of a struggle for Paleo eaters. No grain implies no sandwiches, a big favorite for lunchtime.

There are no worries, here are some lunch recipes from Paleo that are simple enough to cook up on a Sunday and pack for lunch on a weekday.

# 1. Egg Roll Bowls

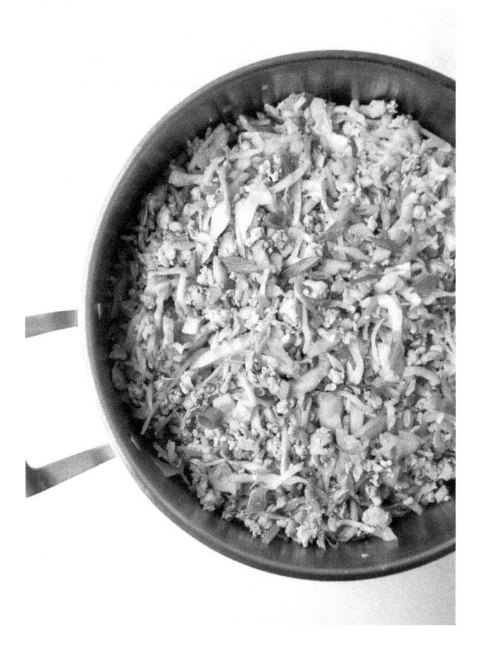

Prep time: 5 minutes

Cook time: 10 minutes.

Total time: 15 minutes

Servings: 6

**Ingredients**

- 1 lb. pork or ground chicken

- 1 teaspoon grated ginger

- 1 teaspoon coconut oil

- 1/3 cup coconut aminos

- 1 teaspoon fish sauce

- 1 teaspoon minced garlic

- 1/2 cup diced water chestnuts.

- 1/2 cup diced mushrooms.

- 1 teaspoon sesame oil

- 1 14 oz. shredded carrots and cabbage (coleslaw mix)

- 2 sliced green onions.

## Instructions

1. In a large, deep skillet, heat the coconut oil. Add the ground chicken and cut it into small parts. Cook until there is no pinker.

2. To the pan, add the mushrooms, green onion, chestnuts, and garlic. For 1-2 minutes, cook and stare.

3. Combine coconut amino, fish sauce, sesame oil, and ginger in a small bowl. Whisk thoroughly.

4. Add the mixture to the pan and then mix to combine. Pour the sauce over the mixture and cook it for around 4-5 minutes, stirring regularly. Slaw has to be wilted but should still have a bit of a crunch.

5. Garnish with green onions and serve.

## 2. Paleo Taco Skillets and Bowls

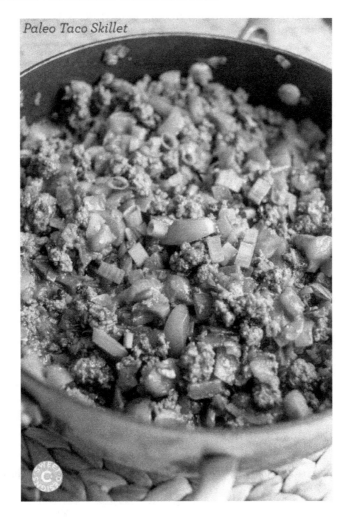

*Paleo Taco Skillet*

Prep time: 5 minutes

Cook time: 15 minutes

Total time: 20 minutes

Servings: 5

**Ingredients**

- 1 diced large onion

- 1 lb. chicken or lean ground beef or turkey

- 1 can green chilies and diced tomatoes

- 2 diced large bell peppers.

- 3 cups greens mix and baby kale or any other salad.

- Taco seasoning

## Instructions

1. Add the ground meat, scramble, and brown in a large skillet.

2. Drain out the extra fat.

3. Add the onion and diced peppers and cook until tender and browned.

4. Add and stir the tomatoes.

5. Mix in the taco seasoning- If required, add a tablespoon of water to mix.

6. Keep on the burner before the taco mix has tacos fully mixed.

7. In a bowl, add the greens or salads and spoon the taco mixture over the end.

8. Enjoy your tacos.

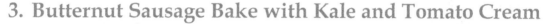

## 3. Butternut Sausage Bake with Kale and Tomato Cream

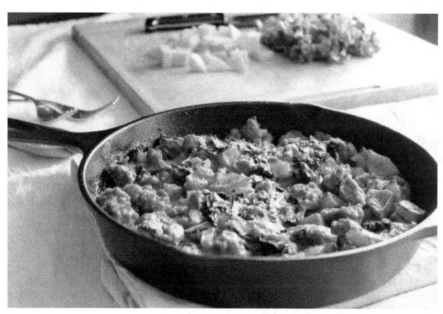

Prep Time: 10 minutes

Cook Time: 1 hour

Total Time: 1-hour 10minutes

Servings: 4 -6 servings

## Ingredients

- 1 tbsp lightly flavored olive oil

- 3 1/2 cups cubed butternut squash.

- 1 lb. Italian pork sausage

- 1/4 tsp fine grain sea salt

- 1/8 tsp crushed red pepper flakes

- 1-2 tsp lightly flavored olive oil

- 1/2 cup marinara sauce (without sugar)

- 1/2 chopped medium onion.

- 2 cups roughly chopped kale

- 1/4 cup full fat canned coconut milk

- Pepper and fine grain sea salt for taste

- 1 whisked egg

## Instructions

1. Roast your butternut squash first. Preheat the oven to 400 degrees F and add one tablespoon olive oil and 1/4 tsp of fine grain sea salt to the butternut squash cubes in a large bowl.

2. in a single layer, Spread the butternut squash cubes on a large baking sheet - or two if necessary - lined with parchment paper. Roast for 30 minutes in the preheated oven, stirring in the middle, until golden brown.

3. Heat a large cast-iron skillet, or another heavy skillet over medium heat while the butternut squash roasts and add 1 tsp of olive oil.

4. In the pan, crumble the sausage and sprinkle it with crushed red pepper. Cook until mostly browned, stirring and breaking up lumps.

5.  Add the chopped onion once the sausage is almost browned and continue cooking until the onion gets soft and the sausage is browned completely.

6.  Next, add the coconut milk and marinara sauce and stir. Bring it to a boil, then bring the heat down to a simmer. To soften, add the kale to the skillet and stir it into the mixture. Remove the skillet from the heat once the kale is tender.

7.  Remove from the oven when the butternut squash is fried, then toss in with the sausage mixture. If you use an oven-proof skillet, everything in it will be baked. If not, then before proceeding, shift the mixture to a greased baking dish.

8.  To the mixture, add the whisked egg and toss gently to combine. Bake for 20-30 minutes in a preheated oven until toasty browned and set.

9.  Before serving, let it sit for 10 minutes. Keep leftovers preserved for up to 3 days in the refrigerator. Enjoy!

## 4. Dutch Oven Grecian Chicken

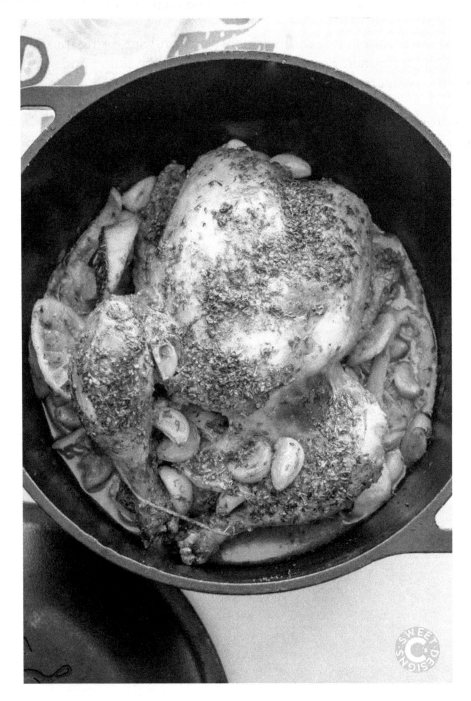

Prep time: 10 minutes

Cook time: 1 hour 30 minutes.

Additional time: 10 minutes

total time: 1 hour 50 minutes

Servings: 8

## Ingredients

- 2 sliced lemons

- whole chicken

- 1 tbsp dried oregano

- 3/4 cup peeled garlic

- 1-2 pats of butter, (optional)

- Pepper and salt

## INSTRUCTIONS

1. Preheat the oven to 375 degrees F.

2. With 5-8 garlic cloves, stuff half lemon into the cavity of the chicken.

3. Sprinkle a good quantity of salt and pepper on chicken.

4. Toss the rest of the lemon and garlic in the Dutch oven.

5. Sprinkle the oregano on the chicken.

6. Add a pat or two of butter on the top if you want the extra crispy chicken meat.

7. Cover with lid and cook for 1 1/2 hours, checking the temperature after an hour for every 20 minutes. You have to get to 160 degrees and then remove the lidded Dutch oven to achieve the safe temperature of 165 ° F for a chicken, as it will keep cooking.

8. After removing from the oven, let the Dutch oven sit for 10 minutes to allow cooking for carryover, so the juices have a rest.

9. Remove from the pan and enjoy your meal.

## 5. Snappy Italian Sweet Potato Spaghetti Bowls

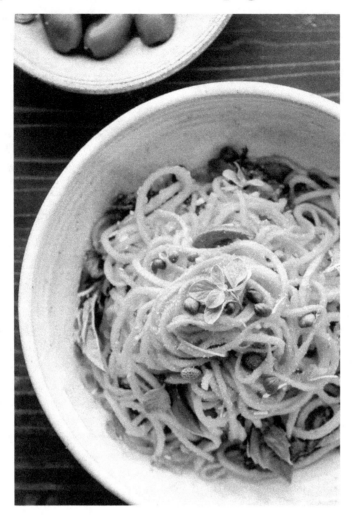

Prep Time: 10 minutes

Cook Time: 10 minutes

Total Time: 20 minutes

Servings: 3 medium servings or 2 large servings

### Ingredients

- 1 tsp minced garlic

- 2 peeled sweet potatoes.

- 1 tbsp avocado oil or vegan butter

- 1/4 cup chopped onion.

- Sea salt

- 1/2 tsp pepper

- 1/2 cup fresh spinach or kale

- 1 tsp red chili pepper flakes

- 14.5 Ounce can have crushed tomatoes or diced tomatoes.

For the tomato sauce:

- 3 marinated artichoke hearts

- 2 peeled garlic cloves

- 1/4 tsp pepper and salt

For topping:

- 1–2 tbsp capers

- A handful of black olives

- A handful of fresh herbs. You can take oregano and basil.

**Instructions**

1. Peel the sweet potatoes first and then spiral them out into noodles. If you do not have a spiralizer, you may cut them and make something of a "stir fry" with julienne.

2. Chop the onion and mince the garlic as well.

3. First, put 1 tbsp of water in a microwave-safe bowl of sweet potato spaghetti noodles.

4. Put in a high microwave for approximately 30-40 seconds to soften. Put aside.

For the Sauce:

1. Put all the rest of your sauce ingredients in a food processor or blender, then drain your tomatoes.

2. Blend until completely smooth.

Assembling the dish

1. In a big pot, skillet, or pan, put your onion, garlic, and oil/butter. Fry until fragrant and softened with onion for 1 -2 minutes.

2. Mix your tomato sauce and let it cook on medium for another minute or so.

3. Finally, add kale or spinach, spaghetti noodles, and the rest of your spices/seasoning to your sweet potato.

4. Toss and cook on medium or until the spinach/kale is softened and the noodles are cooked to your liking for around 8-10 minutes. Every couple of minutes, keep tossing the noodles with the other ingredients.

5. Finally, add the olives and capers and toss them again. You can also wait for your olives and capers to be added to each bowl.

6. Serve in bowls, then cover each bowl with any extra tomato sauce from the pan.

7. Add Salt and pepper for taste.

8. You can keep these for 5 days in fridge.

## 6. One Pan Balsamic Chicken And Veggies

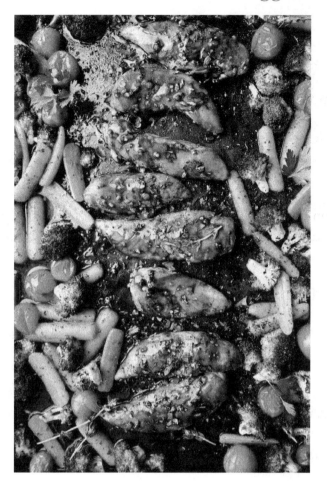

Prep time: 10 minutes

Cook time: 20 minutes.

Total time: 30 minutes

Servings: 4

**Ingredients**

- 1/2 cup fat free zesty Italian dressing

- 6 tablespoons balsamic vinegar

- 2 heads broccoli

- 1.25 pounds chicken breasts or tenders

- 1/2-pint cherry tomatoes

- 1 cup baby carrots

- 3 tablespoons olive oil

- 1 teaspoon Italian seasoning

- Fresh parsley, pepper, and salt (optional)

- 1/2 teaspoon garlic powder

**Instructions**

1.      1. Preheat the oven to 400°F. Spray a wide tray with nonstick spray (line with parchment paper if your tray is not already nonstick or it would stick to the Italian+balsamic mixture) and put it aside.

2.      2. Whisk the zesty Italian dressing and balsamic vinegar together.

3.      3. Trim the fat tenderloins and undesired components. Alternatively, cut the breasts into small pieces that are a 1/4th-1/2nd inch thick.

4.      4. In a wide sack, put 1/3 cup of the Italian+balsamic mixture and add the chicken tenders. Coat and marinate for at least 30 minutes and up to 6 hours in the refrigerator.

5.      5. In little bits, chop the broccoli. Slice the carrots in two.

6.      6. Put broccoli + carrots with cherry tomatoes on the prepared tray. Add olive oil, Italian seasoning, seasoned salt, garlic powder, and pepper to taste.

7.      7. For 10-15 minutes, roast the vegetables.

8.      8. Remove from the oven. Section each side of the tray with the veggies and put the chicken tenders in the middle. Brush over the chicken with 1/3 cup Italian+balsamic mixture.

9.      9. Return to the oven and roast, depending on the chicken size, for another 7-15 minutes. Be cautious about tracking the chicken so it does not overcook. The cooking time will vary according to the size of your chicken.

10.     10. Serve your chicken and vegetables with the remaining Italian+Balsamic mixture. If needed, top with freshly chopped parsley.

11.     Serve with quinoa or rice.

# 7. Paleo Skillet Beef Fajitas

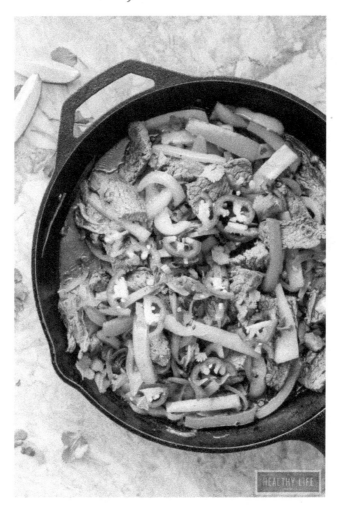

Prep Time: 8 minutes

Cook Time: 22 minutes

Total Time: 30 minutes

Servings:  6

**Ingredients**

Steak:

- 1 juiced lime

- 1 1/2 lb. sliced into thin ribbons flank steak.

- ¼ teaspoon ground cayenne red pepper

- ½ teaspoon chili powder

- 1/8 teaspoon paprika

- 1/8 teaspoon cumin

- ½ teaspoon dried oregano

- 1/8 teaspoon ground black pepper

- 1/4 teaspoon ground black pepper

- ½ teaspoon Sea salt

Vegetables:

- 1 yellow bell pepper de-seeded, trimmed, and sliced.

- 2 tablespoon organic coconut oil

- 1 yellow onion peeled, trimmed, and sliced into thin slices.

- 1 red bell pepper de-seeded, trimmed and sliced.

- 5 ounces shitake mushrooms

- 1 minced garlic clove

- 1 cup vegetable broth

- 2 sliced green onions.

- 1/4 cup chopped cilantro.

- 1 seeded jalapeno sliced thinly.

- 1 avocado seeded, peeled and thinly sliced.

## Instructions

1. Place lime juice, steak, and spices in a big bowl and toss until the steak is coated evenly. Put aside.

2. Over a medium-high flame, put a big heavy skillet. You can use cast-iron.  Add the steak and coconut oil to the skillet when it is melted.

3. Try to set out the steak to be in the skillet in a single layer.

4. Let the steak sear for 3-4 minutes, flip and cook for an extra 3-4 minutes on the other side of the steak, ensuring that the outside is fully seared. Take the steak out of the skillet and put it aside on a platter.

5. Add onions, garlic, peppers, and mushrooms to pan, flipping to coat. To toss and coat your veggies, there should be some juice from the steak. If not, add about a quarter of a cup of the vegetable broth. Try to scrape some extra brown bits that are sticking to the bottom of the plate. Toss your vegetables before they start to soften, around 5 minutes. Combine the green onion, vegetable broth, jalapeño, steak, and any juices on the tray.

6. For an additional 5-8 minutes, toss and cook.

7. Toss cilantro on top and additional jalapeño slices and sliced avocado if you wish. Remove from the flame.

8. Serve with cups of rice, fajitas, or lettuce.

# Chapter 5: Dinner Recipes

the Paleo Diet called the Stone Age Diet had obtained a misleading reputation for being uber-restrictive over the years, forcing individuals to cut out every carb and meat.

Yet, following Paleo is more than converting into a strict carnivore meal plan. The paleo diet is mostly about avoiding highly processed and sugar-loaded food.

So, for dinner, no grains, dairy, or legumes. But yeah, for meat, for poultry, for seafood, for vegetables, for fruit, for nuts. To enjoy the Paleo diet, the following dinner recipes are all you need.

## 1. Easy Paleo Turkey Meatballs with Apples & Savory Herbs

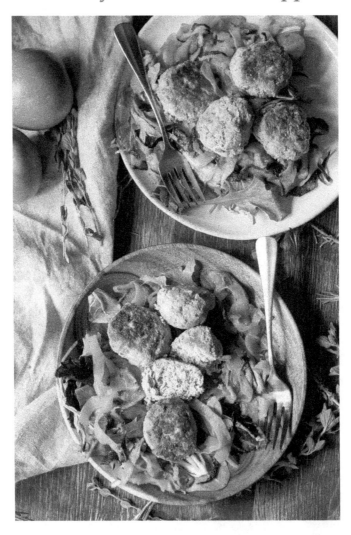

Prep Time: 5 minutes

Cook Time: 15 minutes

Total Time: 20 minutes

Servings: 4 servings

## Ingredients

- 1 medium apple peeled and grated or shredded.

- 1.25 lbs. ground turkey (85-94% lean)

- 2 tbsp almond flour

- 1 egg

- 1 Tbsp finely chopped fresh thyme.

- 1 Tbsp finely chopped fresh rosemary.

- 1/2 tsp fine grain sea salt

- 1/2 Tbsp finely chopped fresh sage leaves.

- 1 tbsp coconut oil for frying

- black pepper for taste

## Instructions

1. Preheat the oven to 400 degrees F and get the meatballs ready for cooking with a large oven-proof skillet.

2. Combine all the ingredients in a wide mixing bowl and combine with your hands to spread them equally, but do not overwork the meat.

3. Preheat the medium-high heat to your oven-proof skillet and add the coconut oil. Form the mixture of turkey into 13-14 meatballs and add them to the heated skillet. Allow them to get brown for 5 minutes on all sides, turning when needed.

4. Transfer the skillet to your preheated oven after the meatballs are browned and bake for about ten more minutes until the juices are cooked and clear. Remove from the oven and serve with your favorite veggie noodles, more fresh herbs for garnish, or potatoes. Enjoy!

## 2. Paleo Creamy Basil & Tomato Chicken

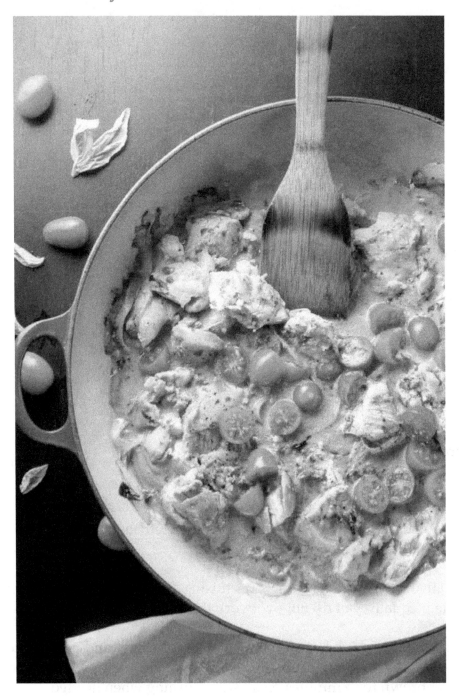

Prep time: 5 minutes

Cook Time: 25 minutes

Total Time: 30 minutes

Servings: 4

**Ingredients:**

- 1/2 yellow onion

- 1-pound skinless boneless chicken breasts or thighs

- 1/2 teaspoon arrowroot powder

- 1 teaspoon coconut oil

- 1/2 cup canned coconut milk

- 1/3 cup cold water

- 1 cup sliced cherry tomatoes.

- 1 batch dairy-free nut-free pesto

**Nut-Free Dairy-Free Pesto:**

- 2 tablespoons sunflower seeds

- 3 garlic cloves

- Salt & Pepper

- 1 tablespoon nutritional yeast

- 1 tablespoon avocado oil

- 1 package fresh basil (2/3 oz)

**Instructions:**

1. 1. Preparing the pesto: put the garlic in a food processor bowl. Pulse until finely minced with the garlic. Add sunflower seeds and pulse several times. Add a dash of pepper, a pinch of salt and the nutritional yeast to the food processor. Finally, add the avocado oil and basil. Pulse until it is well minced with the basil. Place aside the pesto as you cook the rest of the dish.

2. 2. In a large skillet on medium heat, heat the coconut oil until it sizzles. When the oil heats, slice the onion into strips and then add it to the skillet. Cook till they are translucent.

3. 3. Add the chicken to the pan when the onion gets translucent. Cook for 12 minutes, flip over, and cook for an extra 13 minutes. The chicken should be cooked. If it is not, continue cooking until there is no pink in the center of the chicken, and the juices are clear.

4. 4. Stir the arrowroot powder in water in a medium bowl. Add the coconut milk, and then mix in the pesto. Pour the sauce along with the chicken into the skillet. Then bring it to a slight simmer.

5. Add the cherry tomatoes. Simmer for another 1-2 minutes, until the tomatoes are hot, and serve.

6. Serve over spiralized sweet potatoes or zoodles.

## 3. Grilled Teriyaki Salmon Bowls

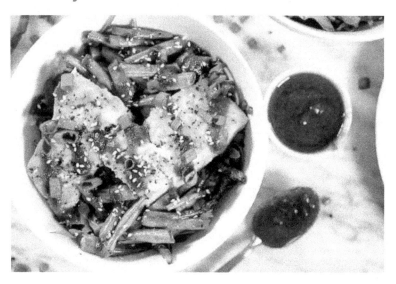

Prep Time: 10 minutes

Cook Time: 15 minutes

Total Time: 25 minutes

Servings: 2

**Ingredients**

- 4 fillets salmon

FOR THE TERIYAKI SAUCE:

- 2 dates pitted and soaked for 10-15 minutes in warm water then drained.

- 1/2 cup coconut aminos

- 1 tsp fresh grated ginger

- 1.5 tsp apple cider vinegar

- 1 tsp garlic powder

FOR THE REST OF THE BOWLS:

- 1/2 bunch bottoms trimmed asparagus and cut into pieces of 1 inch.

- 1 lb. trimmed green beans.

- Sea salt and pepper

- 1 tbsp avocado oil

- 1 cup white rice or cauliflower rice

- 4 cups greens

- 1 tsp sesame seeds

- 1/4 cup chopped green onion.

## Instructions

1. Heat the grill over medium-high heat and grease. Heat up to 400 ° Fahrenheit on a Traeger.

2. Cut the vegetables and put them in a pan on the grill. Drizzle with some avocado oil and season to taste with sea salt and black pepper. Then set aside.

3. In a food processor or blender, put all of the sauce ingredients and process continuously to mix all the ingredients until smooth. Stop for scraping down the sides as required and restart.

4. Put the sauce in a medium saucepan and heat over low heat as the rest of the meal is prepared, stirring regularly.

5. Season the salmon with salt and black pepper and put the flesh on the grill. Grill it for 8 minutes and flip it carefully. Cook for another 6 minutes until the salmon is cooked. Add the vegetables at the same time as the salmon to the grill. When turning the salmon, toss them around.

6. Heat the cauliflower rice after you flip your salmon (or white rice). For cooking cauliflower rice, heat it with a little oil in a skillet and season with salt and pepper to taste.

7. When the salmon is cooked, gently remove the grilled salmon and vegetables.

8. Have your bowls assembled. Make a base of cauliflower, greens, or white rice, the veggies, salmon, and drizzle with sauce. Add sesame seeds and green onion to garnish. Enjoy!

## 4. Lemon Rosemary Chicken Recipe

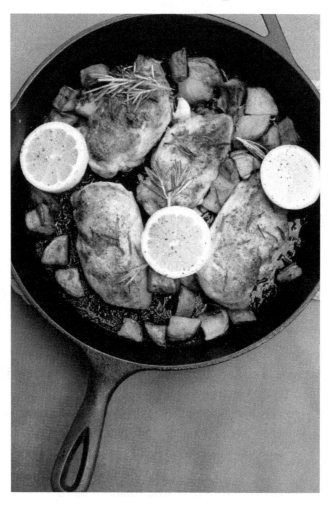

Prep Time: 10 minutes

Cook Time: 60 minutes

Total Time: 1 hour 10 minutes

Servings: 4

**Ingredients**

- 4 chicken breasts

- 1/4 cup olive oil

- 1 squeezed large lemon.

- 1 1/2 cubed sweet potatoes.

- 2 Tablespoons rosemary

- 1 sliced large lemon

- Salt and pepper for taste

- 5 crushed garlic cloves

## Instructions

1. To 400 degrees F preheat the oven.

2. In a large roasting pan or cast-iron skillet, add olive oil and cook over medium-high heat. You may need to do it on two stoves if you use a roasting pan.

3. Sprinkle the chicken breasts with the desired quantity of salt and pepper. Then put the sides of the chicken breast in the pan. Add the chunks of sweet potatoes and cook for 4-5 minutes in a pan or skillet just until the chicken gets golden brown.

4. Turn the chicken over. Then pour rosemary, lemon, and garlic on the potatoes and chicken. Top with some sliced lemons.

5. Bake for 30-35 minutes at 400 degrees until the chicken is cooked.

# 5. Paleo Thai Chicken Pineapple Curry

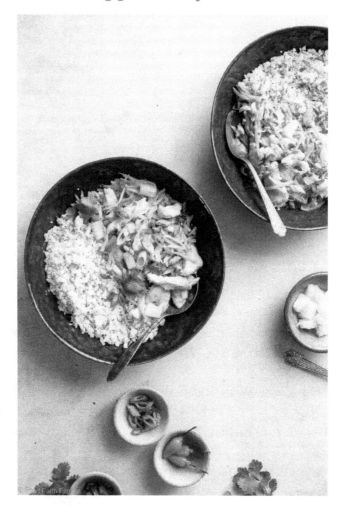

Prep Time:5 minutes

Cook Time: 15 minutes

Total Time: 20 minutes

Servings: 2

**Ingredients**

- 6 tablespoons Pineapple Juice

- 2/3 cup Full Fat Coconut Milk

- 2 cups Cauliflower cut into small bite sized florets.

- 2 teaspoons Yellow Curry Paste

- 1/3 cup Pineapple Tidbits

- Sea Salt

- Sliced Green Onions, for garnishing

- Fresh Cilantro, for garnishing

## Instructions

1. Heat 1 teaspoon of coconut oil over medium/high heat in a wide skillet. Add the chicken breast and cook for about 5 minutes until it gets golden brown.

2. Add the ginger and broccoli slaw and cook until it starts to soften, around 1 minute, in another 1 tsp of coconut oil.

3. Add the pineapple juice, milk, and curry paste to the coconut milk. Lower the heat to medium and put it to a simmer. Simmer for one minute, lower the heat to medium and simmer for around 10-12 minutes, stirring regularly, until thick and reduced.

4. In a food processor, put the cauliflower and cook until it is "rice-like."

5. Heat the last teaspoon of coconut oil over medium/high heat in a medium saucepan. Cook the cauliflower rice, stirring regularly, until golden brown.

6. Divide the curry into two bowls until it has thickened, accompanied by the pineapple tidbits and rice.

7. Garnish with cilantro and green onion.

# 6. Paleo Pineapple Fried Rice

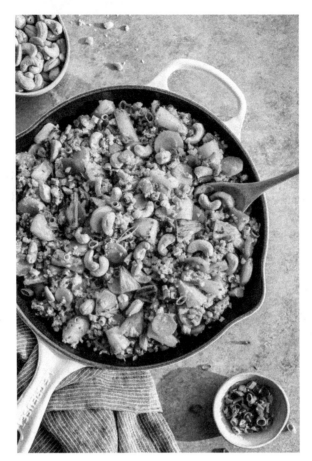

Prep Time: 30 minutes

Cook Time: 10 minutes

Total Time: 40 minutes

Yield: 6 servings

**Ingredients**

- 1/2 lb. skinless boneless chicken thighs cut into small bite sized chunks.

- 1/4 cup avocado oil

- 1 red bell pepper cut into 1/2″ pieces.

- 2 cups small chunks of fresh pineapple (8 ounces)

- 2 cloves minced garlic.

- 4 small thinly sliced carrots (8 ounces) or (2 cups)

- 1 cauliflower (1 lb. 11 oz), or you can get 5 cups frozen cauliflower rice.

- 1 bunch of thinly sliced green onions.

- 4 eggs

Sauce:

- 1/4 cup of coconut aminos

- 1/2 teaspoon chili paste, or you can use 2 teaspoons red pepper flakes.

For finishing:

- Sea salt for taste

- 1 cup roasted cashew pieces

**Instructions**

1. Before you begin cooking, begin by planning all your ingredients since this dish comes together easily.

2. Grate the cauliflower and put it aside using a box grater. Or, when using frozen cauliflower rice, skip this stage.

3. Crack the eggs into a bowl and whisk them gently with a fork.

4. In a small bowl, mix the chili paste or red pepper flakes and coconut amino and set aside.

5. Preheat a very wide non-stick skillet for a few minutes over medium-high heat until it is hot but not smoking.

6. Put one tablespoon of avocado oil in the pan and golden brown the pieces of chicken. Take them out of the pan and put them aside.

7. Then add the pineapple carefully, add one more tablespoon of oil to the pan.

8. Sear the chunks of pineapple to make 2-3 minutes of caramelized edges. Remove and set aside the pineapple from the pan as you finish the fried rice.

9. Add to the pan the remaining two tablespoons of avocado oil and sauté the carrots, bell pepper, and garlic until the vegetables are soft and crisp. Then add cauliflower rice and green onions to the pan.

10. Cook for around 1-2 minutes just until the cauliflower is soft. Add the eggs and cook for 1-2 minutes, stirring until the egg scrambles around the stir-fry.

11. In the pan, add the sauce and cook for another 1-2 minutes before the sauce is fully absorbed and blended.

12. Stir in the chicken, cashews, and caramelized pineapple and remove the fried rice from the flame. Taste test to see if you like any sea salt to be added and serve instantly!

13. This stir-fry tastes hot best but also nice at room temperature.

## 7. One Skillet Tilapia Veracruz

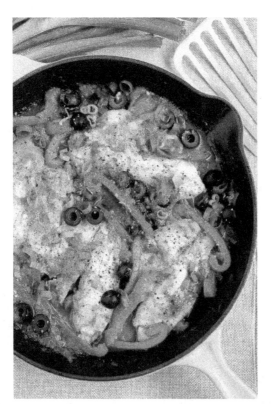

Prep Time: *10* minutes

Cook Time: *20* minutes

Total Time: *30* minutes

Servings: 1

**Ingredients**

- 2 chopped tomatoes

- 3 Tbsp extra virgin olive oil

- 1 thinly sliced medium onion

- 1 thinly sliced red bell pepper

- 3 minced garlic cloves

- 1/2 cup tomato sauce

- 1 Tbsp rinsed and drained capers

- 1/2 cup halved and pitted black pitted olives,

- 1/4 cup white wine

- 1 Tbsp chopped jalapeño pepper slices

- salt and ground black pepper for taste.

- 1 Tbsp oregano

- 4 tilapia filets

## Instructions

1. Heat the oil on a medium-high flame in a large skillet. Add bell peppers, diced tomatoes, and sliced onions. Season and stir with salt. Reduce the heat to medium, cover with a lid and steam until the vegetables are tender, around 3-4 minutes.

2. Add the tomato sauce, olives, minced garlic, capers, white wine, and jalapeno peppers. With freshly ground pepper, salt, and oregano, season again. Stir well.

3. Season with freshly ground black pepper and salt on both sides of the tilapia filet and put-on top of the Veracruz sauce. Spoon the tilapia filets' top with some sauce. Cover with a cap and proceed to cook for around 5 to 6 minutes over medium heat on the stove until the fish flakes easily with a fork.

# Chapter 6: Kids friendly recipes

Here's a collection of recipes that every kid will enjoy! There are some recipes in there that have a little spice in them, but to match your child's needs, you can easily lower that spice down. These recipes would not only keep your kids satisfied and full but also keep you guys amused for a short period between DIY projects and games.

## 1. Breakfast Bacon And Maple Meatballs

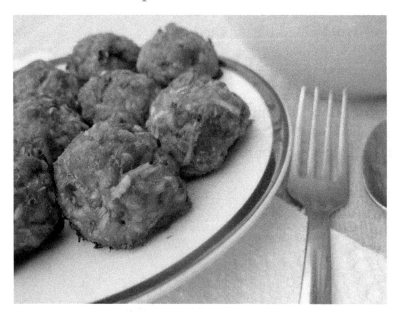

Prep Time: 10 minutes

Cook Time: 35 minutes.

Total Time: 45 minutes

Servings: 4

**Ingredients**

1. 1 sweet potato

2. 1lb breakfast sausage

3. ½ peeled yellow onion.

4. 4oz button mushrooms

5. 2 tablespoons of maple syrup

6. 1 minced garlic clove

7. 5–6 slices of bacon

8. salt and pepper for taste

**Instructions**

1. Preheat the oven to 375°F.

2. Place your slices of bacon over medium heat in a pan. Cook until crispy on all sides, put on a paper towel to soak up and cool the excess fat, then dice up into tiny parts that will fit in meatballs well.

3. Put the sweet potato in a food processor with the shredding extension. Shred your sweet potato, cut its parts, then shred it again. It should be pretty fine.

4. Then, cut the onion and mushrooms with the already shredded sweet potato in the same bowl.

5. Along with your maple syrup, breakfast sausage, diced bacon, garlic clove, salt, and pepper, add the mushrooms, sweet potato, and yellow onion to a bowl and combine well.

6. Then begin making the meatballs and place parchment paper on a baking sheet.

7. Roll your hands on the scooped balls and put them on a baking sheet. Repeat till you have all the ingredients gone.

8. Bake for 30-35 minutes until the meatballs are fully cooked and golden brown. Make sure to check one meatball before you turn off the oven!

9. Pair your breakfast meatballs with some almond milk and serve.

## 2. Breakfast Fries

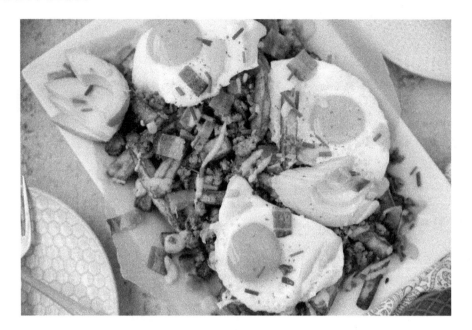

Prep Time: 15 minutes

Cook Time: 1 hour 15 minutes

Total Time: 1 hour 30 minutes

Servings: 4-6

**Ingredients**

- 2lb Yukon gold potatoes cut into fry slices (you can also use sweet or white potato).

- 1/2lb bacon

- 2–3 tablespoons of avocado oil

- 4 eggs (or more depending upon servings)

- 1 lb. breakfast sausage

- 1/2 thinly sliced avocado

- 1/3 cup cheese (dairy-free)

- salt and pepper, for taste

- 1 tablespoon fresh chives, chopped.

## Instructions

1. Preheat the oven to 375° F. Line an aluminum foil baking sheet, then put a wire rack on its top. Spray the wire rack with some avocado oil, put pieces of bacon flat on the wire rack and bake in the oven for around 20 minutes until slightly crispy. Then set it aside to cut into pieces. Leave the oven on.

2. Slice the potatoes into fry slices as the bacon is cooking, sprinkle with salt and toss in the avocado oil. Put the basket in an air fryer without overcrowding and cook for 15-18 minutes at 390 degrees F, tossing after every 4-5 minutes till the potatoes get crispy.

3. Put a wide nonstick sauté pan over medium flame as the potatoes are frying, add breakfast sausage, cut into tiny chunks, and cook until no pink remains, around 10 minutes. Then put it aside.

4. Turn down the heat to low in the hot pan with the left fat (about 2-3 tablespoons). Crack four eggs in the pan and cook until the whites are cooked, and the yolks are still runny about 5-7 minutes.

5. In the microwave or a saucepan, heat the dairy-free cheese until it gets warm.

6. In the wire rack, add the fries and top it with the crumbled bacon and breakfast sausage and put in the oven to bake for 5 minutes and ensure that it is at the same temperature.

7. top it with eggs, sliced avocado, dairy-free cheese, chives, and a sprinkle of pepper and salt to taste.

## 3. Pizza Fries

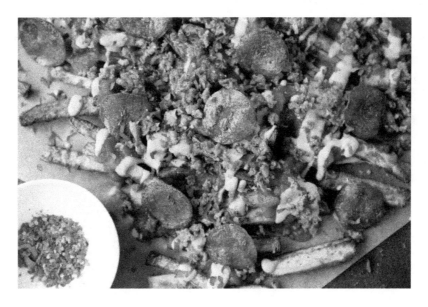

Prep Time: 10 minutes

Total Time: 10 minutes

Servings: 2-3

## Ingredients

- 2–3 tablespoons avocado oil

- 4 Yukon gold potatoes cut into fry slices (you can also use sweet or white potatoes)

- 1/2 lb. hot Italian sausage

- Pinch of salt

- 1/4–1/3 cup pizza sauce

- 10–15 pepperoni slices

- parsley, for garnishing

- 1/4–1/3 cup cheese (dairy-free)

- red pepper flakes, for garnishing

## Instructions

1. Cut the potatoes into strips, add the avocado oil and sprinkle with salt. Put the basket in an air fryer without overcrowding and cook for 15-18 minutes at 390 degrees F, flipping every 4-5 minutes until the potatoes are crispy.

2. Add the Italian sausage to a large non-stick pan as the potatoes are cooking and cut into pieces, cooking until golden brown and no pink remains. Take out from the pan and set aside. Add the pepperoni to the pan and cook the pepperoni on each side for 1-2 minutes.

3. In the microwave or sauté pan, heat the pizza sauce and dairy-free cheese until it gets warm.

4. Top with parsley, Italian sausage, pizza sauce, pepperoni, dairy-free cheese, and red pepper flakes when the potatoes are done cooking.

# 4. Pizza Egg Bites

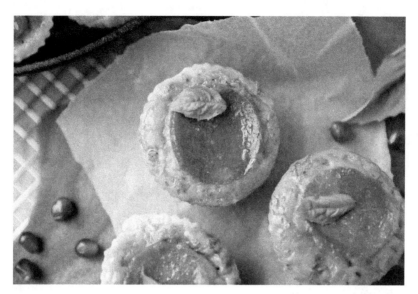

Prep Time: 10 minutes

Cook Time: 45 minutes

Total Time: 55 minutes

Servings: 16-18 egg cups

## Ingredients

- 1/2 minced yellow onion.

- 1/2 lb. Italian sausage

- 1 cup pizza sauce

- 2 minced garlic cloves

- salt and pepper, for taste

- 1 tablespoon chopped fresh basil.

- 8 eggs

- 16–18 pepperoni slices

## Instructions

1. Preheat the oven to 350°F. To make sure nothing sticks, line 2 muffin tins with 16-18 silicone muffin liners and coat them with coconut oil spray.

2. Cook Italian sausage with onion and garlic in a pan over medium flame, cutting the sausage into tiny chunks until golden brown and cooked through.

3. In a large bowl, add the Italian sausage, and add the basil, pizza sauce, salt, and black pepper. Mix and combine. Then add eight cracked eggs to the bowl and mix them one more time to combine thoroughly.

4. In the muffin cup, pour the mixture into 16-18 cups, leaving a little space so the eggs can bubble up as they are baking. Top each muffin cup with a pepperoni slice and put it in the oven to bake for 30-35 minutes until it is baked from the middle.

5. Then all you have to do is pack these muffins and enjoy them throughout the week.

# 5. Strawberries Cream Collagen Shake

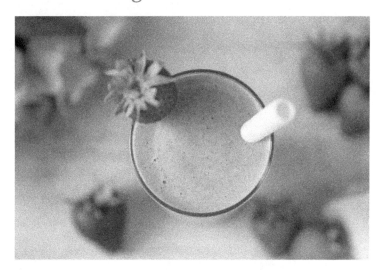

Prep Time: 5 minutes

Total Time: 5 minutes

Servings: 1

## Ingredients

- 1 cup almond milk

- 1 1/2 cups frozen strawberries

- 1 tablespoon maple syrup

- 1/3 cup canned coconut milk

- 1 scoop (10g) collagen peptides

## Instructions

1. Put all the ingredients in a cup blender.

2. Blend until combined and smooth.

3. Enjoy.

# 6.Cookie Dough Collagen Bars

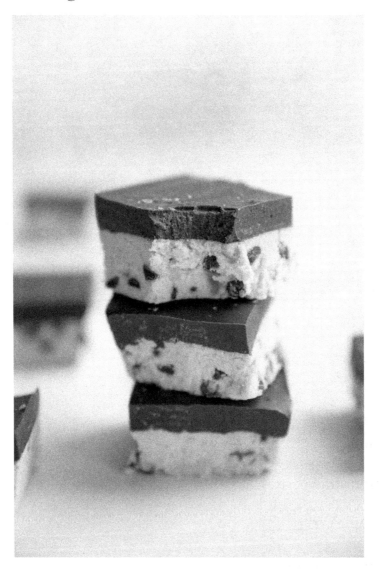

Prep Time: 20 minutes

Total Time: 1 hour 20 minutes

Servings: 8-10 bars

## Ingredients

- 1/2 cup maple sugar

- 1/2 cup ghee or softened coconut oil or grass-fed butter

- 1/4 cup collagen peptides

- 1 teaspoon vanilla extract

- pinch of salt

- 1/2 cup cassava flour

- 1/2 cup mini chocolate chips

For the chocolate layer

- 1/4 cup cashew butter

- 1 cup chocolate chips

- coarse salt

**Instructions**

With parchment paper, line a 9×5 loaf pan.

2. Cream together sugar softened coconut oil (butter or ghee) and vanilla extract until mixed, using a stand mixer or hand mixer.

3. Add the collagen peptides slowly, then add the cassava flour as the mixer spins until all the flour is mixed. Then add in the chocolate chips and salt. In the loaf pan, put the cookie dough, spread around, then press down equally throughout. Set it in the refrigerator.

4. In a double boiler or the oven, melt the cashew butter and chocolate chips until smooth and softened. On top of the cookie dough layer, pour chocolate, spread thinly throughout, and dust on top with coarse salt. Place for 1 hour or longer in the refrigerator to set.

5. for 5-10 minutes, set this loaf pan on the countertop before removing it from the pan right before serving. Then under hot water, run a sharp knife, dry it, and slice into 8-10 squares. All you have to do now is feed yourself! Store it in the refrigerator.

# 7. Chocolate Chip Pancake Bites

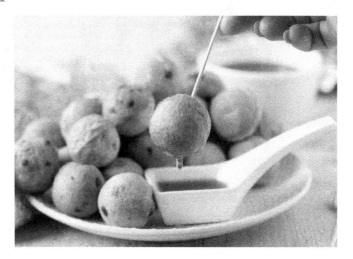

Prep Time: 10 minutes

Cook Time: 15 minutes

Total Time: 25 minutes

Servings: 30-32 pancake bites

## Ingredients

- 1 cup almond milk

- 3 whisked eggs

- 1 teaspoon vanilla extract

- 1 tablespoon maple syrup

- 1/2 cup tapioca flour

- 1/2 cup coconut flour

- 1/2 teaspoon baking soda

- 1/2 teaspoon baking powder

- 1/2 cup mini chocolate chips

- pinch of salt

- maple syrup, for dipping

- coconut oil spray

**Instructions**

1. Heat the Cake Pop Maker.

2. Mix the wet ingredients eggs, maple, almond milk, and vanilla extract in a big bowl.

3. Then add the coconut flour, a pinch of salt, baking powder, tapioca flour, and baking soda. Whisk until the batter is combined properly. Finally, add the chocolate chips and fully mix them up.

4. Use Coconut Oil Spray to grease the Cake Pop Maker. Use a tablespoon or cookie scoop to fill any round of cake pop (be careful that you do not overfill). Follow the cake pop maker's directions to bake until each pancake bit is baked through. Repeat until no batter is left—30-32 pancake bites should be made!

5. Serve with maple syrup!

# 8.Cinnamon Sugar Pumpkin Doughnut Holes

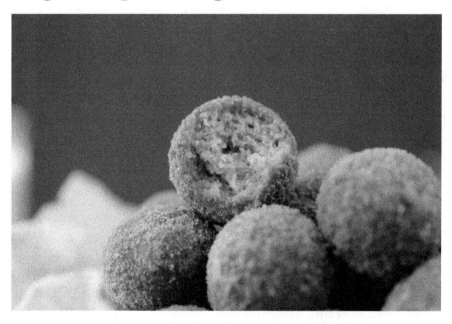

Prep Time:15 minutes

Cook Time: 15 minutes

Total Time: 30 minutes

Servings: 16-19 donut holes

## Ingredients

- 1/3 cup maple syrup

- 1/3 cup pumpkin puree

- 2 whisked eggs.

- 3 tablespoons melted ghee.

- 1 1/2 cups almond flour

- 1 teaspoon pumpkin pie spice

- 3 tablespoons tapioca flour

- 1/2 teaspoon baking soda

- 1/2 teaspoon baking powder

- 1 teaspoon vanilla extract

- pinch of salt

For the cinnamon sugar topping

- 1/3 cup coconut sugar

- 1/4 cup melted ghee.

- 1/2 teaspoon pumpkin pie spice

## Instructions

1. Preheat your mini donut maker.

2. In a wide bowl, put the eggs, pumpkin, ghee, maple syrup, granulated sugar, and whisk until smooth and mixed. Then add almond flour, tapioca flour, baking soda and baking powder, pumpkin pie spice, and salt and mix until smooth.

3. Use a coconut oil spray to grease the donut maker. To scoop the mixture into each donut mold, use a cookie scoop. Follow mini donut maker instructions and cook however suggested. Repeat until you have all the batter is filled in molds. This is expected to make around 16-19 donuts.

4. Place the melted ghee in a small bowl and coconut sugar in another small bowl with pumpkin pie spice. In the molten ghee, dip each donut hole and put in the coconut sugar. Then toss until fully coated. Repeat for all the donuts. Eat up quickly while the donuts are still warm!

## 9. Peanut Butter and Jelly Overnight Chia Pudding

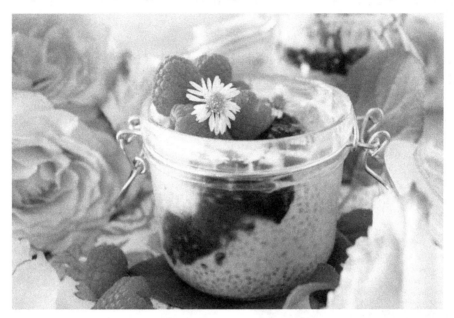

Prep Time: 5 minutes

Refrigerating 12 hours

Total Time: 12 hours

Servings: 2-4

**Ingredients**

- 1/3 cup sunflower seed butter

- 1 cup almond milk

- 1 teaspoon vanilla extract

- 1/4 cup maple syrup

- 1/2 cup raspberry jam

- 1/4 cup chia seeds

- 1 cup raspberries

**Instructions**

1. In a high-speed mixer, blend the almond milk, maple syrup, sunflower seed butter, and vanilla extract until combined.

2. Put the blended mixture into a big resealable jar and add the chia seeds. Seal the jar and shake well.

3. Put in the fridge for about 30 minutes and shake again. This would keep the chia seeds from being separated from the fluid. Then put it back overnight or at least 3+ hours in the fridge.

4. Mix in some raspberry jam the next day and also top it with fresh raspberries!

## 10. Peanut Butter and Jelly Smoothie Bowl

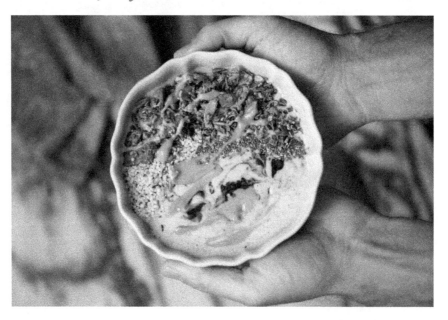

Prep Time: 5 minutes

Total Time: 5 minutes

Servings: 1

**Ingredients**

For the smoothie

- 1 cup almond milk

- 1 frozen banana

- 2 tablespoons raspberry jam

- 3 tablespoons sunflower seed butter (you can use any other nut butter)

- 1 tablespoon ground chia seeds

- 2 tablespoons unflavored collagen peptides

- 1 tablespoon maple syrup

- 1 tablespoon flaxseed meal

- 1 teaspoon vanilla extract

For the toppings:

- 1 tablespoon sunflower seed butter (you can use another nut butter)

- 1/4 cup paleo granola

- 2 teaspoons cacao nibs

- 1 tablespoon raspberry jam

- 1/2 teaspoon chia seeds

- 1 teaspoon hemp heart

**Instructions**

1. Put all the smoothie ingredients in a blender and blend till combined and smooth.

2. Pour the smoothie into a bowl.

3. Top your smoothie with the topping ingredients.

4. Enjoy.

# 11.Blueberry Orange Pancakes

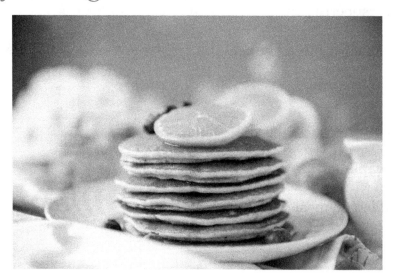

Prep Time: 10 minutes

Cook Time: 15 minutes

Total Time: 25 minutes

Servings: 8-10 pancakes

## Ingredients

- 2 whisked eggs.

- 1 cup almond milk Greek yogurt

- 3 tablespoons orange juice

- zest of 2 oranges

- 1 teaspoon vanilla extract

- 2 tablespoons maple syrup

- 1 cup almond flour

- 1 cup tapioca flour

- pinch of salt

- 1 teaspoon baking powder

- 1 cup blueberries (some more for garnishing)

## Instructions

1. In a large bowl, whisk together the maple syrup, yogurt, eggs, zest, orange juice, and vanilla extract.

2. Mix in the tapioca flour, almond flour, baking powder and some salt. Then fold in the blueberries.

3. Put the pan on the stove on medium heat, grease the pan, and scoop the batter into the pan using an ice cream scoop. Cook for 2-3 minutes on each side, till bubbles start appearing in the batter, then flip.

4. Top the pancakes with syrup and blueberries.

5.

# Conclusion

Paleo diet is one of the most trendy weight loss diet plans, but it is grounded in the food patterns of our ancestors from tens of thousands of years ago. A paleo diet is targeted at shifting to a form of life that is much like what early humans consumed. The rationale of the diet is that the human body is mismatched genetically with the diets that are practiced in the todays world that originated with agricultural activities, an idea known as discordance.

Compared with other dietary plans, such as the Diabetes Diet or the Mediterranean Diet, various clinical trials have compared the paleo diet. Overall, these findings indicate that when compared with vegetables, fruits, lean meats, legumes, whole grains, and low-fat dairy items, a paleo diet can have certain advantages. Those advantages may include:

- Lower triglycerides

- More reduction of weight

- Strengthened tolerance to glucose

- Improved regulation over blood pressure

- Better management of appetite

Considering its benefits, paleo is recommended for giving a go with the provided recipes for at least 30 days.

# THE 5-INGREDIENT PALEO DIET COOKBOOK

Cook and Taste Tens of Easy Paleo Recipes to Raise Body Energy and Balance Blood Glucose

By

Chef John Tank

## Table of Contents

# Introduction

Life runs at warp speed these days and, when it comes to cooking and eating, healthy habits usually fall short. We make quick decisions and opt for unhealthy choices when, in reality, eating bad food will do more harm to our bodies than good. That's why my 5-Ingredient Paleo Cookbook can be the answer to your prayers. With just 5 simple ingredients that only a mother could love, you can make life-changing recipes and provide your family with a new, fresh start to life.

You'll be happily surprised at how easy it is to make delicious, nutrient-dense foods that will get your family off their skinny pedestals and onto the carousel of health by restoring their taste buds to something more savory and healthy.

What are the Benefits of the 5-Ingredient Paleo Diet?

The 5-Ingredient Paleo Diet is a simple cookbook with more than 50 healthy, delicious recipes that have been proofed and tested by several bakers and ingredient experts, including chefs and nutritional therapists.

With this simple book, I'm so confident that you can have the most delicious, nutrient-dense foods, I'm even willing to give you my word of encouragement. I'll follow through on my promise that by following my 5-Ingredient Paleo Diet, which has proven to be a delicious way to naturally reduce the disease risk of 50 out of 100 Americans, you will become healthier and more vital!

5-Ingredient Paleo Recipes

Tasty, healthy, and made with only 5 ingredients that won't cost you a dime and set you back five bucks, these recipes have been made with love and my intention is to improve the overall health of every American.

The main purpose of this book is to prove that you don't need a cookbook full of exotic foods and pricey ingredients to make your life better or any changes to your health. Â The 5-Ingredient Paleo Cookbook contains only delicious recipes and provides a boost of energy and nutrients with the minimum amount of effort. If you are someone who is looking for a change in your life, whether it might be a bigger curvy booty, higher metabolism, or you just can't seem to find a good doctor, then this cookbook is the answer to your state-of-mind

## The Rules of Eating Paleo

The Paleo diet has certain guidelines; once you get the hang of these, the plan is easy to follow.

*A PALEO DIET SHOULD BE HIGH IN ANIMAL PROTEIN.* Opt for grass-fed, pasture-raised, or locally sourced animals as often as possible, and look for ethically raised protein sources if at all possible. Meat that comes from nonlocal sources is typically pumped with high amounts of additives such as soy and wheat. The animals are often also treated unfairly and kept in inhumane conditions.

*A PALEO DIET SHOULD BE HIGH IN SATURATED FATS, SUCH AS COCONUT OIL, BUTTER, GHEE, AND ANIMAL FATS.* Eating good fat is good for you! Healthy fats help maintain a healthy heart as well as a lower body fat percentage.

*A PALEO DIET SHOULD HAVE GENEROUS AMOUNTS OF FRESH VEGETABLES.* Organic is always best, but not always possible. Follow the **Dirty Dozen** guidelines when deciding whether to buy organic versus non-organic veggies and fruits. For example, you don't need to buy organic avocados or bananas because you aren't eating the skin, and cauliflower and broccoli are sprayed with fewer pesticides than other vegetables. However, always buy tomatoes and strawberries as organic because they are sprayed with the most pesticides. When choosing fruits, opt for low-sugar fruits that are high in antioxidants, such as fresh berries.

*A PALEO DIET ELIMINATES ALL REFINED SUGARS, INCLUDING FRUIT JUICES,* **EXCEPT** *LEMON AND LIME.* Refined sugar spikes your blood glucose levels, which we want to avoid. Eliminating refined sugars will help naturally balance your blood sugar levels.

*A PALEO DIET ELIMINATES ALL DAIRY,* **EXCEPT** *BUTTER.* High amounts of dairy can cause blood sugar spikes as well as many digestive issues.

*AVOID STRESS AND OPT FOR EIGHT HOURS OF SLEEP WHENEVER POSSIBLE.* Stress wreaks havoc on the body; we need sleep to balance our hormones and keep our cortisol levels from spiking throughout the day.

*EXERCISE IS KEY!* Lifting weights and working out has been shown to reduce osteoporosis, certain cancers, and excessive weight gain. Aim for at least 30 minutes of exercise each day.

The recipes in this book will help you lead a healthy, active lifestyle—less time meal planning and shopping mean more time for that walk or workout. Each recipe adheres to the preceding dietary guidelines and will make living a Paleo life easier and more fun. With fresh, simple ingredients in each recipe, I take the thinking out of cooking and the stress out of mealtime! Plus, who doesn't love eating colorful food?

# Chapter 1: Smoothies & Breakfasts

### Veggie Power Smoothie

Prep & Cooking time: 30 minutes
Serves: 2

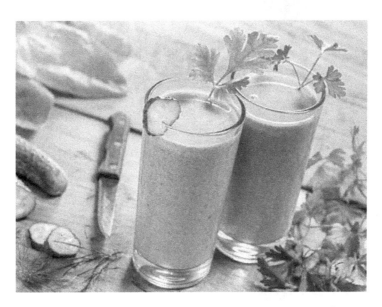

## Ingredients
- 1 cup chopped kale

- ½ cup chopped broccoli

- ½ cup frozen cauliflower

- 1 cup chopped green apple, plus green apple slices, for garnishing (optional)

- 1 cup almond coconut milk

- 1 tablespoon honey (optional)

## Directions
1. In a blender, combine the kale, broccoli, cauliflower, chopped apple, and almond-coconut milk. Blend for 2 to 3 minutes until smooth and creamy.
2. Taste and add the honey (if using) for more sweetness, or omit it for a vegan version.
3. Pour into tall glasses and garnish each with an apple slice, if desired.
Make it easier tip: Prep the ingredients at the beginning of the week and refrigerate in an airtight container. All you need to do is pour the prepped ingredients into a blender and you are ready to go! These can also be made into smoothie packs and stashed in the freezer.
Pro tip: Boil your veggies first, freeze them, and then add them to your smoothies. This helps your body absorb the nutrients from the veggies better and will help you digest everything.

## Pumpkin Pie Smoothie

Prep & Cooking time: 10 minutes
Serves: 2

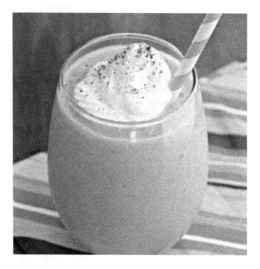

## Ingredients

- 1 cup canned pumpkin purée

- ½ cup pitted dates

- 2 scoops collagen peptides

- 1 tablespoon honey

- 1 cup almond coconut milk

- 1 cup ice cubes

- The ground cinnamon, for garnishing (optional)

- Ground nutmeg, for garnishing (optional)

## Directions

1. In a blender, combine the pumpkin and dates. Blend on high speed for 2 to 3 minutes.
2. Add the collagen peptides, honey, and almond coconut milk. Blend again on high speed for 2 to 3 minutes.
3. Add the ice. Blend on high speed for 2 minutes more. Pour the smoothie into glasses and top with cinnamon and nutmeg (if using).

Make it easier tip: Assemble the ingredients at the beginning of the week and freeze in airtight containers. All you need to do is pour the prepped ingredients into a blender and you are ready to go!

Variation tip: This pie-flavored smoothie is even more delicious when topped with coconut whipped cream.

## Pineapple Mango Dreaming' Smoothie

Prep & Cooking time: 15 minutes

Serves: 2

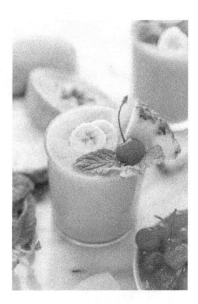

## Ingredients

- 1 cup fresh or frozen chopped mango, plus fresh mango slices, for garnishing (optional)

- 1 cup fresh or frozen cubed pineapple, plus fresh pineapple slices, for garnishing (optional)

- 2 scoops collagen peptides

- ¾ cup pitted dates

- 1 cup almond coconut milk

- 1 cup ice

## Directions

1. In a blender, combine the chopped mango, cubed pineapple, and collagen peptides. Blend on medium speed until creamy. Add the dates and almond-coconut milk. Blend again.

2. Add the ice. Blend everything at high speed for 2 to 3 minutes until smooth. Pour the smoothie into glasses and garnish with fresh mango and fresh pineapple slices (if using).

Variation tip: For an extra-creamy smoothie, combine the almond-coconut milk with the dates and collagen peptides and blend for 2 to 3 minutes until thickened, before adding the pineapple and mango.

### Beets & Berries Smoothie

Prep & Cooking time: 10 minutes
Serves: 2

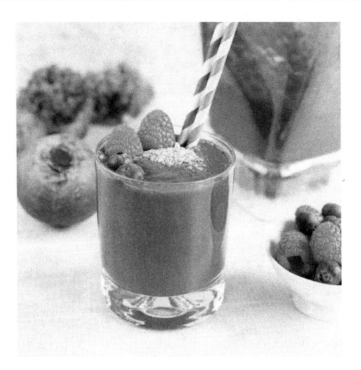

## Ingredients

- 1 cup chopped raw beets

- 1 cup chopped kale

- ½ cup chopped banana

- 1 cup fresh or frozen blueberries, plus more for garnishing (optional)

- 1 cup coconut water

- 1 cup ice

## Directions

1. In a blender, combine the beets, kale, and banana. Blend on low speed to mix.

2. Add the blueberries, coconut water, and ice. Blend on medium speed until smooth and creamy. Pour the smoothie into glasses and garnish with additional blueberries, if desired.

Make it easier tip: Assemble the ingredients at the beginning of the week and freeze in an airtight container. All you need to do is whiz the prepped ingredients in a blender and you are ready to go!


Vanilla Coconut Protein Smoothie

Prep & Cooking time: 10 minutes
Serves: 2 to 3

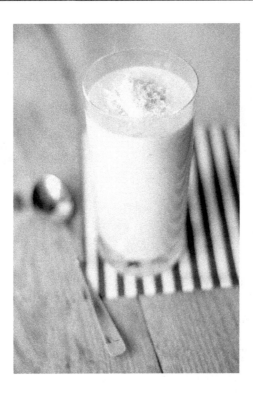

## Ingredients

- 2 cups almond-coconut milk

- 1 cup pitted dates

- 1 tablespoon vanilla extract

- 1 tablespoon ground cinnamon, plus more for garnishing

- 1 cup frozen coconut chunks

## Directions

1. In a blender, combine the almond-coconut milk and dates. Blend on high speed for 1 minute until smooth.
2. Add the vanilla, cinnamon, and frozen coconut chunks. Blend again for 1 minute until smooth and creamy.
3. Pour into glasses and garnish with a sprinkle of cinnamon.
Variation tip: For a different flavor, substitute almond extract for the vanilla.


Ham & Broccoli Egg Cups

Prep & Cooking time: 40 minutes'
Serves: 4 to 6

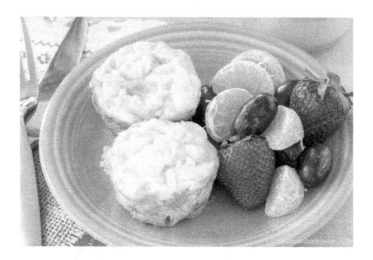

## Ingredients

- 10 slices no-sugar-added ham

- 2 tablespoons coconut oil

- ½ cup chopped bell pepper, any color or a mix

- 1 cup chopped broccoli

- ½ cup almond-coconut milk

- 10 large eggs

- Sea salt

- Freshly ground black pepper

## Directions

1. Preheat the oven to 375°F.
2. Line each well of a muffin tin with 1 slice of ham, forming a cup.
3. In a skillet over medium-high heat, melt the coconut oil. Add the bell pepper. Sauté for 3 minutes until softened.
4. Add the broccoli. Sauté for 5 minutes more until the broccoli begins to soften. Fill the ham cups about half full with the veggies, leaving room for the egg.
5. In a medium bowl, whisk the almond-coconut milk and eggs. Season with sea salt and pepper. Fill each muffin well to the top with the egg mixture. Using a toothpick, stir the veggies and egg together. This step is optional if you are looking for a more layered look to your egg cups.
6. Bake for 20 to 25 minutes until the eggs are set and the cups are slightly browned.
Variation tip: Substitute partially cooked bacon slices for the ham.


Paleo Breakfast Bowl

Prep time: 20 minutes
Serves: 4

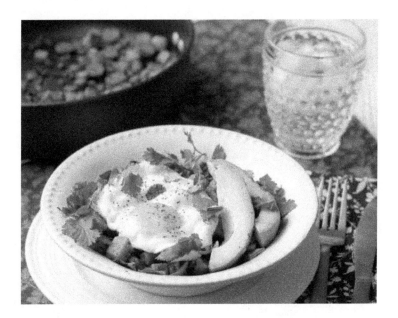

## Ingredients

- 1 cup chopped uncooked bacon

- 2 cups arugula

- 1 cup cherry tomatoes

- 2 avocados, pitted and chopped

- 1 tablespoon coconut oil

- 4 large eggs

- Sea salt

- Freshly ground black pepper

## Directions

1. In a skillet over medium heat, cook the bacon for about 5 minutes until crispy. Transfer to paper towels to drain and cool.

2. Divide the arugula among 4 serving bowls. Top each with cherry tomatoes, chopped bacon, and avocado chunks, placing them in different sections of the bowl.

3. Discard the grease in the skillet, wipe it out, and return it to medium heat. Add the coconut oil.

4. Carefully crack the eggs into the skillet. Fry until cooked to your desired doneness. You may need to fry one or two eggs at a time, depending on the size of your pan. Top each bowl with 1 fried egg, season with sea salt and pepper, and enjoy!

Make it easier tip: Make these salad bowls ahead of time by prepping all the veggies and dividing them among separate bowls. Cook the bacon and eggs on the day you want to eat the salad for breakfast!

Avocado Egg Cups

Prep & Cooking time: 15 minutes
Serves: 4 to 6

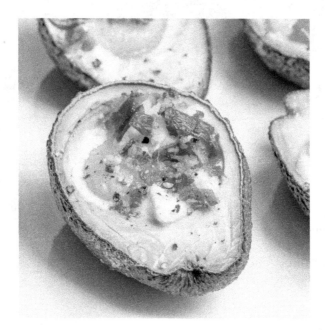

## Ingredients

- 3 avocados, halved lengthwise, pitted, and peeled

- 1 tablespoon freshly squeezed lemon juice

- 1 tablespoon coconut oil

- 6 large eggs

- Sea salt

- Freshly ground black pepper

- 1 cup fresh cilantro, finely chopped

## Directions

1. In a medium bowl, toss the avocados in the lemon juice to keep them from turning brown.
2. In a skillet over medium heat, heat the coconut oil.
3. Carefully crack the eggs into the skillet. Fry until the whites are set. You may need to fry one or two eggs at a time, depending on the size of your pan. Season with sea salt and pepper. Carefully place each cooked egg into an avocado half.
4. Serve the avocado egg cups in ramekins, if desired. Top with cilantro and season again with sea salt and pepper, as desired.
Variation tip: For a different take, you can bake the eggs right in the avocados instead of frying them. Just halve and pit the avocados (don't remove the peel) and scoop out some of the flesh to make room for an egg. Crack the egg into the hole, season with sea salt and pepper, and bake in a 425°F oven for 15 to 20 minutes until the egg is set.

## Oven-Baked Omelets

Prep & Cooking time: 35 minutes
Serves: 4 to 6

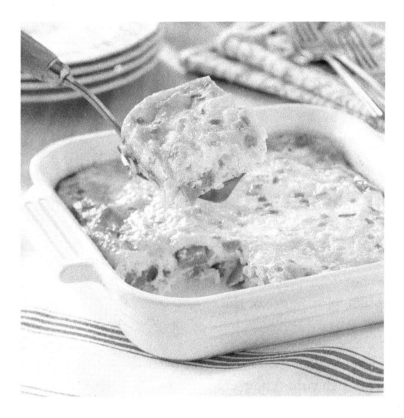

### Ingredients

- 8 large eggs
- 1½ cups almond-coconut milk
- Sea salt
- Freshly ground black pepper
- 2 cups chopped broccoli
- 2 cups fresh spinach
- 1 cup diced tomato
- ½ cup chopped fresh cilantro

### Directions

1. Preheat the oven to 375°F. Coat 4 to 6 ramekins with cooking spray and set aside.
2. In a large bowl, whisk the eggs and almond-coconut milk until combined. Season with sea salt and pepper.
3. Add the broccoli, spinach, and tomato. Stir until well combined. Divide the egg mixture among the prepared ramekins.
4. Place the ramekins on a rimmed baking sheet and transfer to the oven. Bake for about 25 minutes until the eggs are no longer runny and the tops have browned a bit.
5. Serve garnished with fresh cilantro.

*MAKE-AHEAD TIP:* Make a batch of these baked egg cups and stash them in the fridge or freezer. Pop them in the microwave to reheat, or just let them come to room temperature.

## Sweet Potato, Ham & Egg Loaf

*Prep & Cooking time:* 1 hour 10 minutes

Serves: 4 to 6

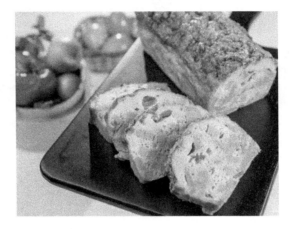

### Ingredients

- 2 tablespoons coconut oil
- 4 medium sweet potatoes, peeled and sliced
- 2 teaspoons paprika, plus more for the eggs
- Sea salt
- Freshly ground black pepper
- 1 medium red onion, sliced
- 2 cups chopped (½-inch cubes) ham
- 10 large eggs

### Directions

1. Preheat the oven to 400°F. Line a 9-by-5-by-3-inch loaf pan with parchment paper. This keeps your loaf from sticking to the pan. Set aside.
2. In a skillet over medium heat, melt the coconut oil. Add the sliced sweet potatoes and season with paprika, sea salt, and pepper. Sauté for 8 to 10 minutes. Add the red onion. Sauté everything for 5 minutes more.
3. Stir in the ham and sauté for 10 minutes. Transfer the sweet potato mixture to the prepared loaf pan.
4. In a large bowl, whisk the eggs. Season with paprika to taste. Slowly pour the eggs onto the sweet potato mixture. Bake for 25 to 30 minutes, or until the eggs are set and everything is nice and crispy.
5. Let cool for 5 minutes before slicing and serving.

*Variation tip:* For added flavor and nutrition, add 1 cup chopped asparagus along with the ham.

## Sheet Pan Breakfast

*Prep & Cooking time:* 35 minutes
Serves: 4 to 6

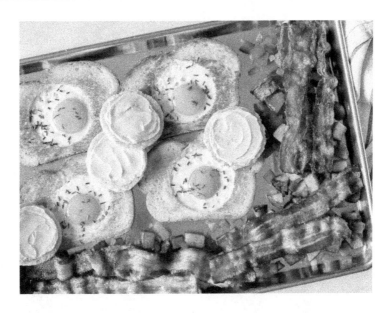

## Ingredients

- Coconut oil spray, for preparing the sheet pan
- 1 cup chopped cauliflower
- 1 cup chopped broccoli
- 1 cup chopped bell pepper, any color or a mix
- ¼ cup EVOO
- Sea salt
- Freshly ground black pepper
- 2 cups ground sausage
- 4 to 6 large eggs (one per person)

## Directions

1. Preheat the oven to 425°F. Coat a sheet pan with coconut oil spray and set it aside.
2. In a large bowl, combine the cauliflower, broccoli, and bell pepper. Pour the EVOO over the veggies and stir to coat. Season with sea salt and pepper. Set the veggies aside.
3. In a skillet over medium heat, cook the sausage for about 5 minutes until just browned. Do not overcook; it will cook more in the oven. Add the veggies and stir to combine. Using a slotted spoon, transfer the sausage-veggie mixture to the sheet pan.
4. Make 4 to 6 holes in the mixture, one hole for each egg.
5. Bake the veggies and sausage for 10 minutes.
6. Remove the sheet pan from the oven. Carefully crack 1 egg into each hole.
7. Bake everything for 5 minutes more, or until the egg whites are set.

Substitution tip: Need a vegetarian option? Easy. Swap the meat for more veggies. Instead of sausage, use Portobello mushrooms and asparagus.

Avocado Egg Sammies

Prep & Cooking time: 15 minutes
Serves: 4 to 6

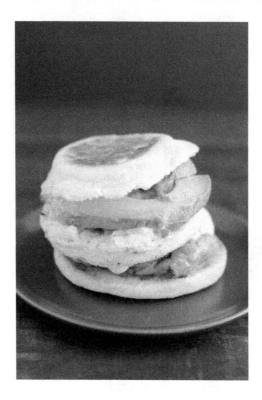

## Ingredients

- 1 (12-ounce) package nitrate-free bacon
- 1 tablespoon ghee
- 4 to 6 large eggs
- 4 to 6 tablespoons Homemade Mayonnaise
- 4 to 6 medium sweet potatoes, baked and halved (see preparation tip)
- 4 to 6 avocados, halved, pitted, peeled, and sliced

## Directions

1. In a skillet over medium-high heat, cook the bacon for about 5 minutes, until crispy. Transfer to paper towels to drain and cool. Once cooled, halve each bacon slice widthwise.
2. In a clean skillet over medium-high heat, heat the ghee.
3. Carefully crack the eggs into the skillet. You may need to fry 1 or 2 eggs at a time, depending on the size of your pan. Fry until the whites are set.
4. Spread 1 tablespoon of mayonnaise on each sweet potato half.
5. Top each half with some avocado slices, bacon slices, and 1 fried egg.
6. Carefully top the egg with the other sweet potato half. You now have breakfast sammies!

Preparation tip: Bake your potatoes beforehand in a 450°F oven for 45 minutes and then slice them in half.

Variation tip: If you are vegetarian, swap the meat for a giant slice of portobello mushroom.

# Chapter 2: Easy Snacks, Appetizers & Sides

### Mini Hamburgers

Prep & Cooking time: 25 minutes
Serves: 4 to 6

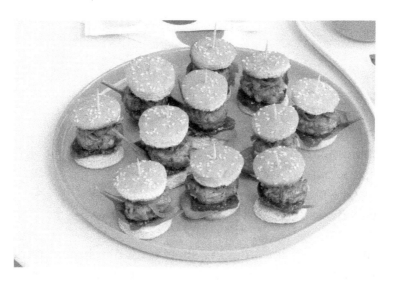

## Ingredients
- 1½ pounds organic ground beef
- ½ medium red onion, chopped
- Sea salt
- Freshly ground black pepper
- 2 cups chopped iceberg lettuce
- 1 cup small pickle chips
- 2 cups cherry tomatoes, halved

## Directions
1. In a medium bowl, mix the ground beef and onion. Season with sea salt and pepper. Gently mix to combine. Shape the beef mixture into mini (1-inch) patties (18 to 20 patties).
2. Heat a grill pan or cast-iron skillet over medium-high heat. When hot, place the patties in the pan. Cook for 2 to 3 minutes per side.
3. To assemble your mini burgers: Top a patty with some lettuce, a pickle, and a tomato half. Insert a toothpick into the mini burger to hold everything together. Repeat this step until you've made all your burgers.

Variation tip: Serve with Simple Ketchup and Homemade Mayonnaise.

### Bacon Jalapeño Poppers

Prep & Cooking time: 40 minutes
Serves: 4 to 6

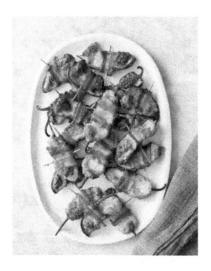

## Ingredients

- 1 (12-ounce) can full-fat coconut cream
- 2 tablespoons chili powder
- 15 jalapeño peppers, halved and seeded
- 15 mini sausages (see tip)
- 15 nitrate-free bacon slices

## Directions

1. Preheat the oven to 425°F. Line a baking sheet with parchment paper and set it aside.
2. In a small bowl, stir together the coconut cream and chili powder until combined.
3. Fill each jalapeño half with about 2 tablespoons of the coconut cream mixture. Reserve the remaining coconut cream mixture for serving.
4. Place a mini sausage on top of each filled jalapeño.
5. Wrap each popper with 1 bacon slice and use a toothpick to secure it, if needed. Place the wrapped jalapeños on the prepared baking sheet.
6. Bake the poppers for 20 to 25 minutes until the bacon is cooked thoroughly.

Ingredient tip: Use nitrate-free bacon and sausages; Applegate makes a great nitrate-free mini sausage.


Mini Pepperoni Pizza Bites

Prep & Cooking time: 25 minutes
Serves: 4 to 6

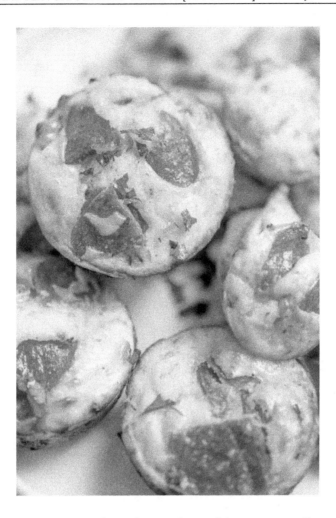

## Ingredients

- 12 slices nitrate-free pepperoni (Applegate brand is very good)
- 2 cups chopped mixed bell peppers
- 1 (4-ounce) can sliced black olives
- 12 whole cherry tomatoes
- 2 cups Paleo Tomato Sauce

## Directions

1. Preheat the oven to 400°F.
2. Press 1 pepperoni slice into each well of a 12-cup muffin tin.
3. Fill each well with bell peppers, olives, and a cherry tomato.
4. Drizzle each pizza bite with about 2 tablespoons of Paleo Tomato Sauce.
5. Bake for 12 to 14 minutes, or until the sauce is bubbling and the pepperoni is nice and crispy.

Variation tip: Garnish with thinly sliced fresh basil leaves for extra flavor and because it makes them look pretty.

### Marinara-Stuffed Mushrooms

Prep & Cooking time: 20 minutes
Serves: 4 to 6

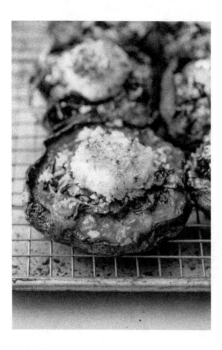

## Ingredients
- 1 (12-ounce) package cremini mushrooms, stemmed
- ¼ cup EVOO
- Sea salt
- Freshly ground black pepper
- 1 tablespoon garlic powder
- 2 cups marinara sauce
- ½ cup chopped fresh parsley
- ½ cup chopped fresh basil

## Directions
1. Brush the mushrooms with EVOO and season with sea salt, pepper, and garlic powder.
2. In a large skillet over medium heat, heat the remaining EVOO.
3. Place the mushrooms in the skillet. Cook for 5 minutes per side, or until tender. Transfer the mushrooms to a glass baking dish, hollow side up.
4. Carefully fill each mushroom with marinara sauce.
5. Top with parsley and basil.
6. If you like them crispy, place the mushrooms in a preheated 350°F oven for 5 minutes.

Variation tip: For a meaty version of this dish, add crumbled cooked sausage (¼ to ½ pound) to the mushrooms before adding the sauce.


### Romaine Lettuce BLT Bites

Prep & Cooking time: 15 minutes
Serves: 4 to 6

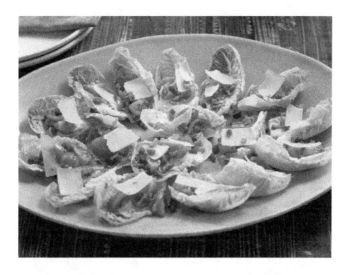

## Ingredients

- 1 (12-ounce) package nitrate-free bacon
- 2 cups sliced mixed tricolor cherry tomatoes
- 6 scallions, white and light green parts minced
- ¼ cup EVOO
- 1 cup freshly squeezed lemon juice
- Sea salt
- Freshly ground black pepper
- 1 head romaine lettuce, leaves separated

## Directions

1. In a skillet over medium-high heat, cook the bacon for about 5 minutes until crispy. Transfer to paper towels to drain. Chop the bacon into small pieces.
2. In a medium bowl, combine the tomatoes, scallions, EVOO, and lemon juice. Season with sea salt and pepper. Gently stir to combine.
3. Fill each romaine lettuce leaf with some of the tomato mixtures.
4. Sprinkle each stuffed romaine leaf with bacon and serve.

Variation tip: Garnish these bites with thinly sliced fresh basil.


### Cauliflower Fried Rice

Prep & Cooking time: 40 minutes
Serves: 4 to 6

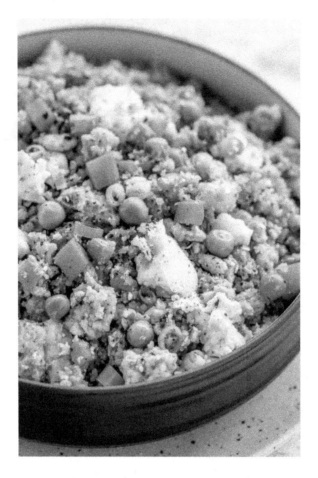

## Ingredients

- 2 tablespoons coconut oil, divided
- 1 pound boneless skinless chicken breast, thinly sliced
- 1 head cauliflower, cut into florets
- 1 tablespoon finely chopped peeled fresh ginger
- 3 large eggs, beaten
- ¼ cup coconut aminos

## Directions

1. In a skillet over medium-high heat, heat 1 tablespoon of coconut oil.
2. Add the chicken. Cook for about 5 minutes until cooked through. Remove from the heat and set it aside.
3. In a food processor, pulse the cauliflower until it resembles rice. Set aside.
4. Heat a large wok or skillet over medium-high heat and add the remaining 1 tablespoon of coconut oil.
5. Add the ginger and sauté until fragrant, about 1 minute.
6. Add the cooked chicken to the wok. Sauté for 3 minutes until heated through.
7. Add the cauliflower rice. Sauté for about 5 minutes until just tender.
8. Add the beaten eggs, scrambling them into the cauliflower.
9. Stir in the coconut aminos. Sauté everything for 5 minutes until browned.

Variation tip: Add 1 cup of shredded carrots and 4 thinly sliced scallions after adding the ginger. Sauté for a few minutes until the carrots begin to soften. Garnish with ½ cup of chopped fresh cilantro.

## Sweet Potato Avocado Cups

Prep & Cooking time: 1 hour 15 minutes
Serves: 4 to 6

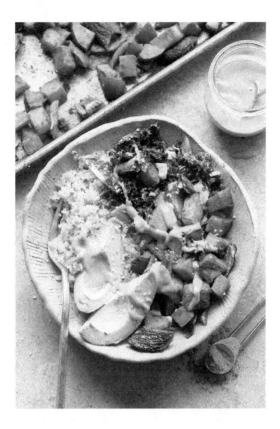

### Ingredients
- 4 sweet potatoes
- 1 tablespoon coconut oil, plus more, warmed, for serving (optional)
- 4 garlic cloves, peeled
- 1 avocado, halved, pitted, and sliced
- 1 cup chopped tomato
- ½ cup chopped red onion
- 1 cup chopped fresh cilantro
- Sea salt
- Freshly ground black pepper

### Directions
1. Preheat the oven to 400°F.
2. Rub each sweet potato with a bit of coconut oil and place on a baking sheet. Wrap the garlic cloves in a piece of aluminum foil and add to the baking sheet.
3. Bake the sweet potatoes and garlic for 1 hour, or until soft. When the potatoes are ready, their skins will peel off easily. Remove and let cool.
4. While the potatoes cook, in a food processor, combine the avocado, tomato, red onion, cilantro, and the roasted garlic cloves (popped from their skins). Pulse for 1 minute.
5. Slice the cooled sweet potatoes down the middle and scoop the avocado mixture into each sweet potato.
6. Season with sea salt and pepper. Drizzle with additional warmed coconut oil, if desired.

Make it easier tip: Instead of baking the sweet potatoes in the oven, cook them in the microwave (place on a microwave-safe plate, poke a few holes in them, and heat on high power for 5 to 10 minutes, until tender). You can also "roast" the garlic in the microwave. Cut the top off a whole, unpeeled head of garlic and place the head in a microwave-safe dish with a bit of water and a drizzle of olive oil. Cover and cook on high power in 2-minute intervals until the garlic is very soft. Squeeze the cooked cloves out of their skins to use.

### Hearty Meatballs

Prep & Cooking time: 55 minutes
Serves: 4 to 6

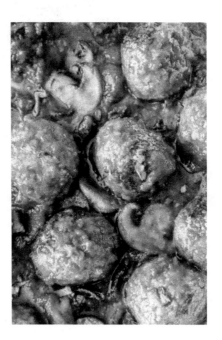

### Ingredients
- 1-pound organic ground beef
- 1 large egg, beaten
- 1 medium red onion, minced
- 2 garlic cloves, minced
- ¼ cup minced fresh parsley, plus additional for garnishing

### Directions
1. Preheat the oven to 400°F. Line a rimmed baking sheet with parchment paper and set it aside.
2. In a large bowl, combine the beef, egg, red onion, garlic, and parsley. Mix, making sure to knead the ingredients together to get the meatball mixture nice and thick. Form the meat mixture into 1-inch balls and place them on the prepared baking sheet.
3. Bake the meatballs for 40 minutes, or until cooked through and no longer pink.
4. Serve the meatballs hot, garnished with parsley.

Variation tip: Serve with Simple Ketchup and Homemade Mayonnaise for dipping.

Roasted Buffalo Cauliflower

Prep & Cooking time: 30 minutes
Serves: 4 to 6

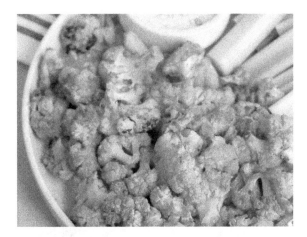

## Ingredients
- 1 head cauliflower, cut into florets
- 3 teaspoons paprika
- 3 teaspoons garlic powder
- 2 teaspoons ground cumin
- Sea salt
- Freshly ground black pepper
- 1 cup freshly squeezed lemon juice
- ½ cup hot sauce (Tessemae's is a great Paleo-friendly brand)
- 2 tablespoons ghee, melted

## Directions
1. Preheat the oven to 425°F. Line a rimmed baking sheet with parchment paper and set it aside.
2. Place the cauliflower in a large bowl and set it aside.
3. In a small bowl, stir together the paprika, garlic powder, and cumin. Season with sea salt and pepper, and stir again to combine.
4. In another small bowl, stir together the lemon juice, hot sauce, and melted ghee. Spread the mixture over the florets.
5. Coat each floret in the spice mixture. Spread the florets evenly on the prepared baking sheet.
6. Bake for 10 to 15 minutes, or until the florets are crispy.

Substitution tip: To make this recipe vegan, substitute coconut oil or olive oil for the ghee.

# Chapter 3: Fish, Beef, Poultry & Seafood Mains

Coconut Chicken

Makes: 6 servings
Prep & Cooking time: 1 hour 5 mins

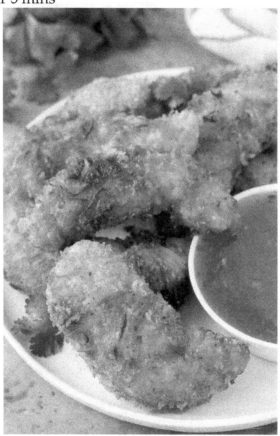

**Ingredients**:
- 1 15-ounce can coconut milk
- 1 whole cut-up chicken
- 2 tablespoons fresh ground ginger
- 6 garlic cloves, minced
- 1/4 cup lime juice
- 1/2 – 1 teaspoon coarse salt
- Fresh chopped cilantro (optional, for garnish)
- 1/2 teaspoon pepper

**Directions**:
1. In a small bowl, whisk lime juice, coconut milk, ginger, garlic, pepper & pepper in a small bowl. Combine marinade and chicken in a big zip-top bag. Let the chicken sit in the marinade for approximately an hour.
2. Preheat oven to 180°C (350°F). Place the chicken in a big baking dish. Bake for about 1 hour – or until the internal temperature of the chicken reaches 165°F.
3. Garnish with cilantro before serving.

Slow Cooker Chicken

Makes: 6 servings
Prep & Cooking time: 6 hours 5 mins

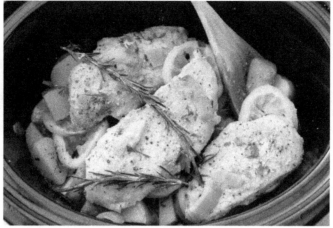

<u>Ingredients</u>:
- 1.5 lbs. skinless, boneless chicken breast (2-3 large)
- 1/2 soy sauce or tamari or coconut aminos
- 1/2 cup sriracha
- 1/2 cup honey
- 2 tablespoons garlic (minced)
- 1.5 tablespoons cornstarch (optional)

<u>Directions</u>:
1. Prepare the sauce first, by whisking together honey, tamari, minced garlic, and sriracha.
2. Add the chicken breasts at the bottom of a slow cooker then pour sauce on top.
3. Adjust the slow cooker to high heat and cook for 2 to 3 hrs. Alternatively set the slow cooker to low and cook for a recommended 6-8 hours.
4. Once the chicken is easy to shred, remove it from the slow cooker and shred the chicken breast using 2 forks.
5. Before you place the shredded chicken back in the slow cooker, add 1.5 tablespoons of cornstarch to thicken the sauce and whisk until adequately dissolved.
6. Add the shredded chicken back in the sauce and stir — air for about 10 minutes before you serve.

Nutritional Facts per Serving: Calories: 231Sugar: 25Fat: 2Carbohydrates: 29Fiber: 1Protein: 27

Chicken Thighs with Balsamic- Raspberry Sauce

Serves: 4
Prep & Cooking time: 30 mins

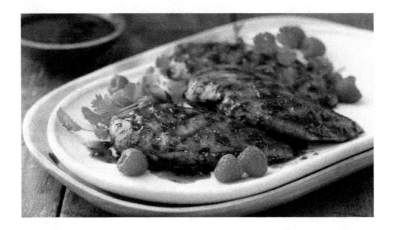

**Ingredients**:
- 1 tablespoon ghee or olive oil
- 4 bone-in skin-on chicken thighs
- Salt, to taste
- Raspberry-Balsamic Sauce:
- 1 cup frozen (thawed) or fresh raspberries
- 1 clove garlic (smashed)
- Optional Pinch dried thyme
- Honey, to taste (optional)
- 1/4 cup aged balsamic vinegar
- Salt, to taste

**Directions**:
1. Preheat oven to 375° Fahrenheit. Pat the chicken thighs to dry and dust liberally with salt. Place a medium-sized oven-safe skillet over medium-high heat. Heat for a few minutes.
2. Add some ghee to the pan. Once the ghee melts, put the chicken thighs in the skillet skin down. Do not touch!! Let it cook for at least 10 minutes or until crispy and golden. Flip the chicken thighs and put the pan in the oven. Allow it to cook for 10 minutes.
3. As the meat cooks, blend the first four ingredients in the blender or food processor. Add salt and honey to taste for those who are not on a whole 30.
4. Remove the pan carefully from the oven after it cooks for ten minutes. Remove the chicken thighs using tongs. Gently remove the chicken from the oven after it has cooked for ten minutes. Remove the thighs from the pan using tongs. Let it rest for 5 minutes on a plate. Serve with balsamic raspberry sauce.

Pulled Chicken

Makes: 6 servings
Prep & Cooking time: 5 hours 5 mins

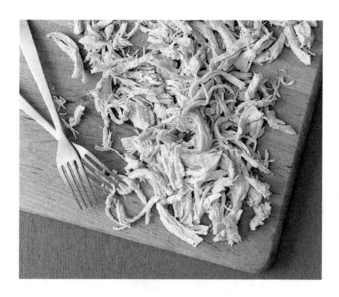

**Ingredients**:
- 2 medium sweet, crisp apples (such as Fuji or Honeycrisp) chopped and cored +
- 1 teaspoon kosher salt
- 1 medium yellow thinly sliced onion
- 1 teaspoon granulated garlic powder
- 2 pounds skinless and boneless, chicken thighs or breasts
- ¾ cup unsweetened apple cider (divided)

**Directions**:
1. Put the onions and apples at the base of a 6-quart slow cooker. Dose with ½ teaspoon salt and toss to combine.
2. Dose both sides of the chicken with an extra ½ teaspoon garlic powder and salt.
3. Put the chicken over the apple and onion mixture. Pour ½ cup apple cider over it and cover to cook for 6 hours on low or 4 hours high or until the chicken cooks through and tender.
4. Take out the chicken and place it on a cutting board. Shred using two forks and place back in the slow cooker. Add the extra ¼ cup apple cider and stir to combine. Taste and add apple cider and salt to taste.


Italian Beef with Zucchini

Serves: 6
Prep & Cooking time: 40 mins

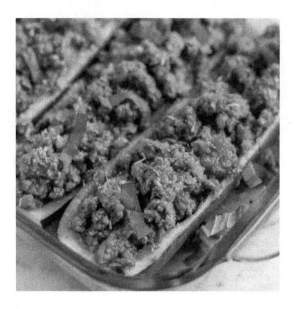

**Ingredients**:
- 3 medium zucchinis (650 grams)
- 1-pound ground beef
- ½ cup diced tomatoes
- 1 ½ cups pasta sauce (divided)
- 1 tablespoon Italian seasoning
- Optional toppings: nutritional yeast, fresh basil, red pepper flakes.

**Directions**
1. Preheat oven to 350F. Pour a ½ cup pasta sauce into a big glass baking dish. Set aside.
2. Make the zucchini boats. Cut the bottom off the zucchini and then slice it in half lengthwise. Remove out the center of the zucchini halves using a spoon and leave about 1/4-1/2 inch shell. Place the zucchini flesh side up in the baking dish.
3. Place a big sauté pan over medium heat. When the pan is hot (approximately 30 seconds) add the ground beef and break it up with a spoon. Sauté it for 4 to 5 minutes until browned. Add in Italian seasoning, diced tomatoes, and a cup of pasta sauce. Stir and remove from heat once properly combined.
4. Divide the beef equally and stuff the zucchini boats (about ½ cup per boat) use foil to cover the pan and bake for 30 minutes or until the zucchini is cooked and a little firm. Garnish with optional toppings. Enjoy!

Nutritional Fact per Serving: Calories from Fat 108, Calories 196, Total Fat 12g 18%, Dietary Fiber 2g 8%, Total Carbohydrates 6g 2%, Protein 16g 32%, Sugars 4g

Turkey Meatballs

Makes: 24 meatballs
Prep & Cooking time: 25 mins

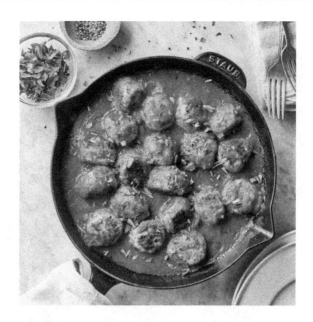

**Ingredients**:
- 1 finely chopped small yellow onion (approx. ½ cup)
- 1 small red bell pepper, orange or yellow bell pepper, thinly chopped (about ½ cup)
- 1 teaspoon garlic powder
- ⅓ Cup almond flour
- ½ teaspoon kosher salt
- 2 tablespoons olive oil
- 1-pound ground turkey (dark or light)

**Directions**:
1. Preheat oven to 400 degrees F.
2. Stir together the bell pepper, onion, garlic powder, flour, and salt in a big bowl. Add turkey and stir again until all the ingredients are properly mixed, but care should be taken not to over mix.
3. Pour 1 tablespoon of olive oil onto a large baking dish or sheet pan. Rub well until the pan is completely coated.
4. Scoop 1 tablespoon of the turkey mixture on your hands and roll it around gently to form a ball. Put the meatball on the oiled pan. Repeat the process with the remaining mixture.
5. Sprinkle the additional 1 tablespoon of olive oil over the meatballs and roll around to properly coat them.
6. Bake the meatballs for approx. 20 minutes, or until they are cooked well and golden brown. Flip once halfway through.


Simple Pork Loin

Makes: 6 servings
Prep & Cooking time: 30 mins

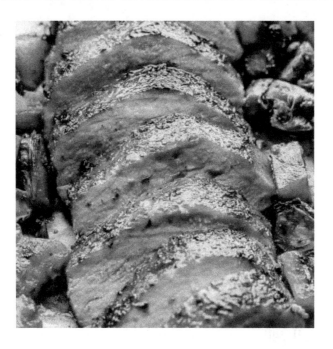

**Ingredients**:
- 1 large onion diced
- 1 ¼ lb Pork Loin seasoned generously with pepper and salt
- 8 oz cherry tomatoes
- 8 cloves garlic diced
- 1 lemon sliced thin

**Directions**:
1. Preheat the oven to 4500.
2. On medium heat, heat a heavy ovenproof pan on the stove.
3. Add pork loin and brown on all sides.
4. Add onions then sauté with pork until browned lightly.
5. Add garlic, tomatoes, and lemon, and heat on high until the tomatoes pop.
6. Move the mixture to the oven and cook until the pork's internal temperature reads 140-155 degrees (depends on how you like your pork).
7. Allow it to sit covered in a pan, for about 8 minutes. This helps the pork's internal temperature to raise an extra 5 degrees and allows the juices to set.
8. Carve and serve. Plate with onions, tomatoes, and garlic from the pan!

Nutritional Facts per Serving: Calories 144, Total Fat 3g 5%,Calories from Fat 27P, Saturated Fat 1g 5%,Sodium 51mg 2%, Cholesterol 59mg 20%, Potassium 478mg 14%, Sugars 1g, Total Carbohydrates 4g 1% , Protein 21g 42%


Slow Cooker Shredded Barbecue Beef

Serves 6
Prep & Cooking time: 7 hours 15 minutes

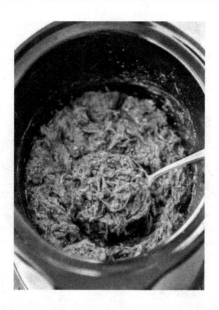

## Ingredients
- 1 (4-pound) pot roast, like bottom round
- ½ cup *Homemade Barbecue Sauce* or bottled barbecue sauce
- ½ cup low-sodium beef broth

## Directions
1. Place the pot roast in a slow cooker and cover with the barbecue sauce and beef broth. Using the back of a wooden spoon or spatula, spread the barbecue sauce over the pot roast. Cover and cook on low for 6 to 8 hours, until a thermometer inserted into the center of the roast reads 145°F.
2. Remove the roast and transfer to a plate, reserving the sauce. Allow the roast to cool for 10 minutes.
3. Using two forks, shred the beef and place into a large bowl. Add the reserved sauce and toss to coat.
4. Serve warm or freeze for later. To freeze, store cooled beef in a freezer-safe container in the freezer for up to 2 months. To defrost, refrigerate overnight. Reheat in a saucepan over medium heat for 5 to 10 minutes, until the beef and sauce are warmed through. Single-serve portions can be reheated in the microwave on high for about 1½ minutes.

Nutritional value Per serving: Calories: 434; Total fat: 13g; Saturated fat: 5g; Protein: 67g; Carbohydrates: 8g; Fiber: 0g; Sodium: 464mg


Slow Cooker Beef with Bell Peppers

Serves 6
Prep & Cooking time: 6 hours 10 minutes

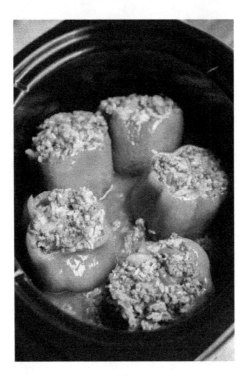

## Ingredients

- 1 (2-pound) top round steak or London broil
- ½ teaspoon salt
- ¼ teaspoon freshly ground black pepper
- 1 large onion, thinly sliced
- 2 red bell peppers, seeded and cut into ¼-inch strips
- ¾ cup *Basic Tomato Sauce* or jarred tomato sauce
- ½ cup low-sodium beef broth

## Directions

1. Season the steak with salt and pepper, and place in the slow cooker. Top with the onion, peppers, tomato sauce, and broth. Stir to combine.
2. Cover and cook on low for 6 to 8 hours, until the beef, reaches an internal cooking temperature of 145°F.
3. Cut the steak into thin slices and serve warm or freeze for later. To freeze, place cooled steak with vegetables and liquid into a reseal able container in the freezer for up to 2 months. To defrost, refrigerate overnight. Reheat in a large skillet on the stovetop for about 10 minutes, or reheat individual portions in the microwave on high for about 2 minutes.

Serving size: 4 ounces steak plus about ½ cup vegetables
Per serving: Calories: 248; Total fat: 9g; Saturated fat: 3g; Protein: 34g; Carbohydrates: 6g; Fiber: 2g; Sodium: 386mg


## Pork Larb

Serves 4
Prep & Cooking time: 25 minutes

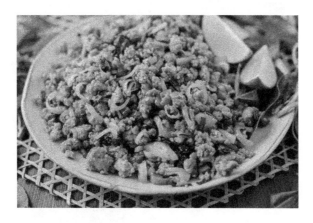

## Ingredients

- 1 tablespoon olive oil
- 1 pound ground pork
- ¼ cup Thai Dressing
- 3 shallots, thinly sliced
- ½ cup chopped fresh cilantro
- 24 Bibb lettuce leaves

## Directions

1. In a medium skillet over medium heat, heat the olive oil. When the oil is shimmering, add the ground pork and cook for 10 to 12 minutes, until browned, using a wooden spoon to break it up. Remove from heat and drain any liquid. Allow the pork to cool for 10 minutes.
2. Pour the Thai Dressing into a medium bowl. Add the cooked pork and toss to blend. Add the shallots and cilantro, and gently stir to incorporate.
3. Scoop 2 tablespoons of the meat into each of 24 lettuce leaves. Serve warm.

Serving size: 6 pieces

Per serving: Calories: 402; Total fat: 33g; Saturated fat: 8g; Protein: 22g; Carbohydrates: 6g; Fiber: 1g; Sodium: 131 mg

Herbed Pork Meatballs

Serves 4
Prep & Cooking time: 30 minutes

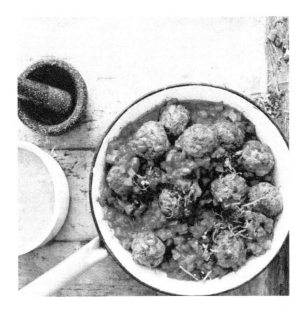

## Ingredients

- 1 pound ground pork
- 1 onion, finely chopped
- 1 garlic clove, minced
- 1 large egg, beaten
- ½ cup whole-wheat panko bread crumbs
- ½ cup finely chopped fresh parsley
- ½ teaspoon salt
- ¼ teaspoon freshly ground black pepper
- 2 tablespoons olive oil

## Directions

1. In a large bowl, combine the ground pork, onion, garlic, egg, bread crumbs, parsley, salt, and pepper.
2. Shape 1 tablespoon of the pork mixture into a ball, and place on a large plate. Repeat with the remaining mixture to make about 20 meatballs.
3. In a large skillet over medium heat, heat the olive oil. When the oil is shimmering, add the meatballs and cook, covered, for about 15 minutes, browning on all sides until a thermometer inserted into a meatball reads 155°F.
4. Serve warm or freeze for later. To freeze, store cooled meatballs in a resealable container in the freezer for up to 2 months. To defrost, refrigerate overnight. Reheat the meatballs in a saucepan along with *Basic Tomato Sauce*: Bring the sauce to a boil, then lower and simmer for 10 to 15 minutes until the meatballs are warmed through. Single-serve portions of meatballs can be reheated in the microwave on high for about 2 minutes.

Serving size: About 5 meatballs
Per serving: Calories: 365; Total fat: 26g; Saturated fat: 7g; Protein: 23g; Carbohydrates: 9g; Fiber: 1g; Sodium: 406mg

## Asian-Spiced Pork Loin

Serves 8
Prep & Cooking time: 50 minutes

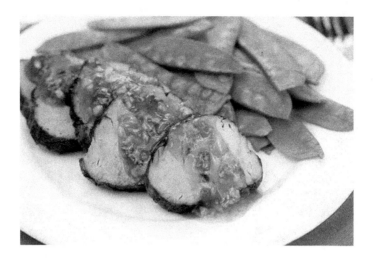

## Ingredients

- ⅓ cup low-sodium soy sauce
- 2 garlic cloves, minced
- 3 tablespoons Chinese five-spice powder
- 2 tablespoons light brown sugar
- 1 teaspoon cayenne pepper
- ½ teaspoon salt
- 1 (2-pound) pork loin, fat trimmed
- Cooking spray

## Directions

1. In a medium bowl, whisk together the soy sauce, garlic, Chinese five-spice powder, brown sugar, cayenne, and salt. Add the pork loin, and turn to evenly coat. Cover the bowl and marinate in the refrigerator for at least 30 minutes or up to overnight.
2. Preheat the oven to 400°F. Coat a baking sheet with cooking spray.
3. Transfer the pork to the baking sheet, discarding the marinade. Bake for 40 to 50 minutes, until a thermometer inserted into the thickest part of the loin reads 145°F.
4. Remove from the oven, and transfer to a cutting board to cool for 10 minutes. Cut into ¾-inch-thick slices.
5. Serve warm or freeze for later. To freeze, store cooled pork in a freezer-safe container in the freezer for up to 2 months. To defrost, refrigerate overnight. Reheat several slices in the microwave on high for 1 to 2 minutes.

Per serving: Calories: 164; Total fat: 5g; Saturated fat: 2g; Protein: 25g; Carbohydrates: 5g; Fiber: 0g; Sodium: 502mg

### Pork Tenderloin with Apple-Tarragon Sauce

Serves 4
Prep & Cooking time: 30 minutes

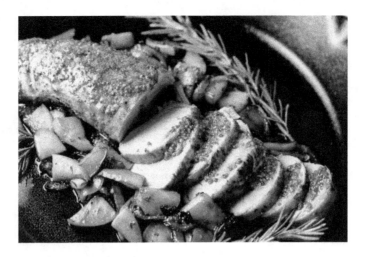

## Ingredients

- 1 tablespoon olive oil
- 1 (1¼-pound) pork tenderloin
- 2 medium apples, cored and sliced
- 1 tablespoon unsalted butter
- 2 garlic cloves, minced
- 2 cups apple cider vinegar
- ½ teaspoon salt
- ⅛ teaspoon freshly ground black pepper
- 2 teaspoons chopped fresh tarragon

## Directions

1. Preheat the oven to 400°F.
2. In a large ovenproof skillet over medium heat, heat the olive oil. When the oil is shimmering, add the pork tenderloin and cook about 8 minutes, turning occasionally, until browned on all sides.
3. Add the apple slices, and place the skillet in the oven. Bake for about 20 minutes, until the pork reaches a minimum internal temperature of 145°F. Place the pork on a cutting board to cool for 5 minutes. Transfer the apples to a plate, and set them aside.
4. Carefully return the skillet to the stovetop over medium heat, and add the butter. When the butter is melted, add the garlic and cook until fragrant, 1 minute. Add the apple cider vinegar, and use a wooden spoon to scrape the pork bits from the bottom of the pan. Bring the mixture to a boil, then reduce heat and simmer for 2 minutes, until the flavors combine. Add the salt, pepper, and tarragon, and stir to incorporate. Turn off the heat.
5. Thinly slice the cooled pork tenderloin, then return it to the skillet. Add the apples and toss to evenly coat. Transfer to a serving dish and serve warm.

Serving size: About 5 ounces pork plus 1¼ cups sauce
Per serving: Calories: 256; Total fat: 9g; Saturated fat: 3g; Protein: 29g; Carbohydrates: 13g; Fiber: 2g; Sodium: 641 mg

Miso-Garlic Pork Chops

Serves 4
Prep & Cooking time: 50 minutes

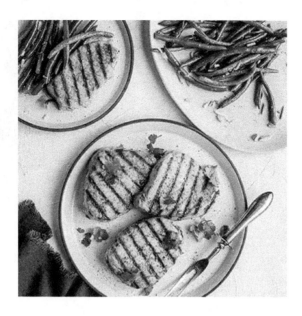

## Ingredients

- ⅓ cup white miso
- ⅓ cup sake
- ⅓ cup mirin
- 2 teaspoons minced fresh ginger
- 1 garlic clove, minced
- 4 (5-ounce) boneless pork loin chops
- Cooking spray, or
- 1 tablespoon olive oil

## Directions

1. In a large bowl, mix the miso, sake, mirin, ginger, and garlic into a smooth paste.
2. Add the pork chops and turn to coat all sides with the glaze. Marinate in the refrigerator for at least 30 minutes or up to overnight.
3. Coat a grill pan with cooking spray and heat over medium heat. Alternatively, brush the grates of an outdoor grill with olive oil. When the pan or grill is hot, cook the pork chops for about 3 to 5 minutes on each side, until they reach an internal cooking temperature of 145°F.

Per serving: Calories: 209; Total fat: 4g; Saturated fat: 1g; Protein: 32g; Carbohydrates: 12g; Fiber: 1g; Sodium: 932mg

Slow Cooker Honey Mustard Pork with Pears

Serves 8
Prep & Cooking time: 4 hours 10 minutes

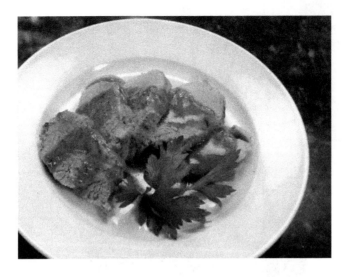

## Ingredients

- ¼ cup Homemade Honey Mustard
- ⅓ cup low-sodium chicken broth
- ½ teaspoon salt
- ¼ teaspoon freshly ground black pepper
- 1 (2-pound) boneless pork loin, fat trimmed
- 2 pears, peeled, cored, and thinly sliced
- 1 tablespoon cornstarch
- 2 tablespoons water

## Directions

1. In a small bowl, whisk together the honey mustard, broth, salt, and pepper.
2. Place the pork and pears in the slow cooker. Pour the honey mustard mixture over the top.
3. Cover and cook on high for 3 to 4 hours or on low for 6 to 8 hours.
4. Remove the pork from the slow cooker, retaining the pears and liquid, and transfer to a cutting board to cool for 10 minutes, then thinly slice.
5. In a small bowl, whisk together the cornstarch and water.
6. In a medium skillet over medium heat, heat the pears and liquid from the slow cooker. Add the cornstarch mixture and continue whisking for about 3 minutes, until the mixture thickens.
7. Serve the pork slices topped with the warm sauce, or freeze for later. To freeze, store cooled pork in a freezer-safe container in the freezer for up to 2 months. To defrost, refrigerate overnight. Reheat in a saucepan over medium heat for 5 to 10 minutes, until the pork and sauce are warmed through. Single-serve portions can be reheated in the microwave on high for about 1½ minutes.

Per serving: Calories: 212; Total fat: 8g; Saturated fat: 2g; Protein: 24g; Carbohydrates: 9g; Fiber: 1g; Sodium: 368mg

Steak Using the Fast-flip Method

Serving: 1

Prep & Cooking time: 5minutes

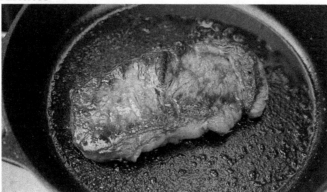

## Ingredients
- 1 beef sirloin steak, at room temperature
- salt to taste
- 3 tbsps. high-heat cooking oil, or as needed

## Direction
1. Set a heavy cast-iron skillet to preheat on medium-high heat. Using paper towels, pat dries the steak on both sides. Season with salt on both sides liberally.
2. Into the hot skillet, drizzle the oil then add the steak and let it cook for 30 seconds. Turn over the steak onto the other side and let it cook for 30 seconds, then turn over again. Keep on turning over, cooking for 30 seconds per side.
3. When it is hot and a bit pink in the middle, starting to firm, and has developed a brown crust, take the steak out of the pan, about 3-4 minutes of total cooking time for an inch of steak. You may check for doneness by using an instant-read thermometer inserted into the middle. Take these numbers as a guideline: 70°C (160°F) for well done, 65°C (145°F) for medium, 54°C (130°F) for medium-rare or 52°C (125°F) for rare.
4. Use two layers of aluminum foil to cover the steak and let it rest for 5 minutes in a warm place.

Nutrition Information: Calories: 645 calories; Total Carbohydrate: 0 g Cholesterol: 98 mg Total Fat: 53.8 g
Protein: 39.3 g Sodium: 237 mg

## Stuffing Meatloaf

Serving: 8
Prep & Cooking time: 60mins

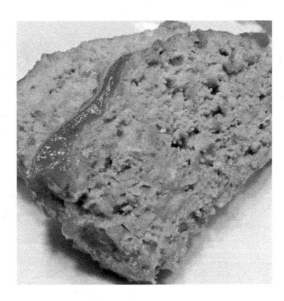

## Ingredients

- cooking spray
- 1 1/2 <u>lbs.</u> ground beef
- 1 small onion, chopped
- 3/4 cup chicken-flavored bread stuffing mix (such as Kraft® Stove Top®)
- 1 egg
- 1 cup shredded mozzarella cheese, or to taste

## Direction

1. Set oven to 375°F (190°C) to preheat. Coat a 9x5-inch loaf pan with cooking spray.
2. In a mixing bowl, combine egg, stuffing mixing, onion, and beef using your hand. Pat beef mixture into the greased pan.
3. Bake meatloaf for 35 to 40 minutes in the preheated oven until the center is no longer pink or an internal temperature of the meatloaf reaches 160°F (70°C) on an instant-read thermometer.
4. Sprinkle shredded mozzarella cheese on top of the meatloaf; allow to sit for approximately 10 minutes or until cheese is melted.

Nutrition Information Calories: 289 calories; Total Carbohydrate: 15.5 g Cholesterol: 83 mg Total Fat: 15.8 g
Protein: 19.9 g Sodium: 430 mg


Stupid Simple Roast Chicken


Serving: 6
Prep & Cooking time: 1 hour 35mins

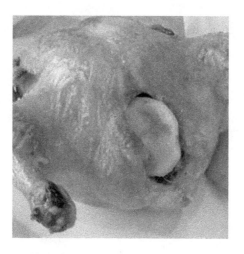

## Ingredients
- 1 (4 lb.) whole chicken, rinsed
- 1 lemon, halved
- kosher salt

## Direction
1. Set the oven to 230°C (450°F) to preheat.
2. In a roasting pan, add chicken and insert it into the cavity with lemon halves, then spread over the outside of the chicken with kosher salt.
3. In the preheated oven, roast chicken for an hour, until juices run clear, the skin is crispy and browned, and an instant-read thermometer reaches 70°C (160°F) after being inserted into the thickest part of a thigh without touching bone. Allow chicken to rest about 15 minutes before carving.

Nutrition Information: Calories: 383 calories; Total Carbohydrate: 2 g Cholesterol: 129 mg Total Fat: 22.8 g
Protein: 41 g Sodium: 1085 mg

## Super Quick Elbows With Tomato Basil Sauce And Cheese

Serving: 2
Prep & Cooking time: 10minutes

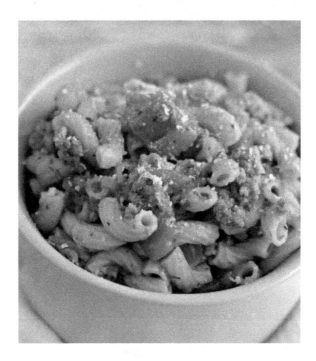

## Ingredients

- 1 pouch Barilla® Ready Pasta Elbows
- 1 cup Barilla® Tomato Basil Sauce
- 2 leaves basil, julienned
- 2 <u>tbsps.</u> Parmigiano-Reggiano cheese, grated

## Direction

1. Rip the edge of Ready Pasta pouch to let air escape. In a microwave, heat for a minute.
2. Warm basil and sauce in a bowl in the microwave for two minutes.
3. Serve pasta with sauce, use cheese to freshen.

Nutrition Information:  Calories: 301 calories; Total Carbohydrate: 56 g Cholesterol: 4 mg Total Fat: 4.4 g
Protein: 10.9 g  Sodium: 696 mg


## Sweet Orange Chicken I

Serving: 4
 Prep & Cooking time: 50mins

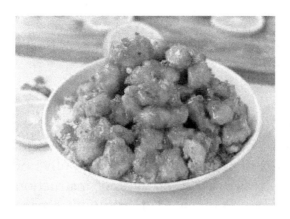

## Ingredients

- 1 (2 to 3 <u>lb.</u>) whole chicken, cut into pieces
- 1/2 cup chutney
- 1/2 cup mayonnaise
- 1/4 cup orange soda
- 3/4 cup water
- 1 <u>tsp.</u> poultry seasoning
- salt to taste

## Direction

1. Set the oven to 175°C or 350°F to preheat.
2. In a 13"x9" baking dish, arrange the chicken pieces. Mix water, soda, mayonnaise and chutney in a moderate-size bowl, then drizzle this mixture over chicken. Use salt and seasoning to sprinkle over chicken.
3. In the preheated oven, bake chicken until it is cooked through and not pink inside anymore, for a half-hour.

Nutrition Information: Calories: 640 calories; Total Carbohydrate: 16.5 g Cholesterol: 151 mg Total Fat: 43.7 g
Protein: 44.3 g Sodium: 296 mg


Tasty Bake Chicken


Serving: 4
Prep & Cooking time: 50mins

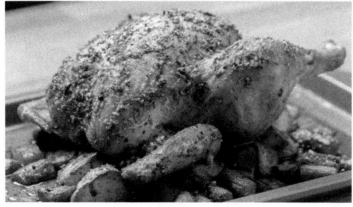

## Ingredients

- 4 chicken breast halves, bone-in
- 1 (.7 <u>oz.</u>) package dry Italian-style salad dressing mix
- 2 <u>tbsps.</u> cold water
- 2 <u>tbsps.</u> olive oil

## Direction

1. Set the oven to 200°C or 400°F to preheat.
2. In a small bowl, pour the entire contents of the salad dressing mix package. Pour in water and mix well together, then stir in olive oil and mix one more time. Do not add in vinegar as directed on package instructions.
3. In a 13"x9" baking dish coated lightly with grease, arrange the chicken breasts with the wrong side facing up, then put on each breast 1/2 tsp. of the dressing mixture and spread out over its surface.
4. Bake at 200°C or 400°F for about 15-25 minutes depending on the breast's size. Flip the breasts over and scoop on the topside the leftover mixture. Bake until juices run clear, chicken is cooked through and tops turn golden brown, about 15 to 20 minutes longer.

Nutrition Information: Calories: 274 calories; Total Carbohydrate: 2.5 g Cholesterol: 82 mg Total Fat: 14.9 g

Protein: 30.1 g Sodium: 864 mg


Tender Flank Steak


Serving: 4
Prep & Cooking time: 8 hours 25mins

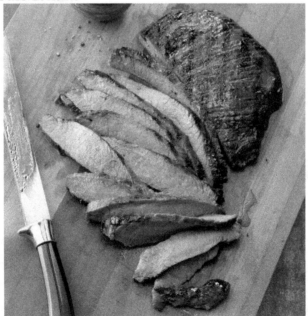

## Ingredients

- 1/4 cup soy sauce
- 1/4 cup Worcestershire sauce
- 1 <u>tbsp.</u> chopped garlic

- 1 (1 <u>lb.</u>) flank steak

## Direction

1. In a bowl, mix garlic, Worcestershire sauce, and soy sauce. Place the mixture in a ziplock bag; add the flank steak and cover with marinade. Press out excess air from the bag; seal. Let it chill in the refrigerator for 8 hrs to overnight.
2. Preheat outdoor grill on medium-high. Grease the grate lightly.
3. Take the steak out of the bag and shake off the excess marinade. Get rid of leftover marinade.
4. Grill steak in the preheated grill for 7 minutes per side until it's hot, starting to get firm, and the center is a bit pink. An inserted thermometer in the middle of the steak should register 60°C or 140°F. Cut the steak against the grain. Serve.

Nutrition Information: Calories: 125 calories; Total Carbohydrate: 5.2 g Cholesterol: 25 mg Total Fat: 4.6 g
Protein: 14.8 g Sodium: 1095 mg

## Tender Slow Cooked Pork Roast

Serving: 8
Prep & Cooking time: 8 hours 20m

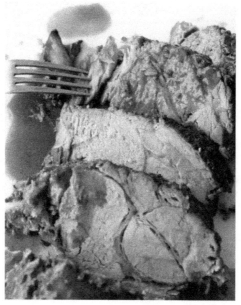

## Ingredients

- 1 (4 <u>lb.</u>) pork shoulder roast
- 1 (8 <u>oz.</u>) can tomato sauce
- 3/4 cup soy sauce
- 1/2 cup white sugar
- 2 <u>tsps.</u> ground mustard

## Direction

1. In a slow cooker, add pork roast. In a bowl, combine together ground mustard, sugar, soy sauce, and tomato sauce while stirring to dissolve sugar. Drizzle the mixture over pork roast, then cook on low setting for 8 hours, until meat is extremely tender.

Nutrition Information: Calories: 362 calories; Total Carbohydrate: 16 g Cholesterol: 89 mg Total Fat: 21.6 g
Protein: 25.2 g Sodium: 1567 mg

### Bacon-Wrapped Shrimp

Prep & Cooking time: 40 minutes
Serves: 4 to 6

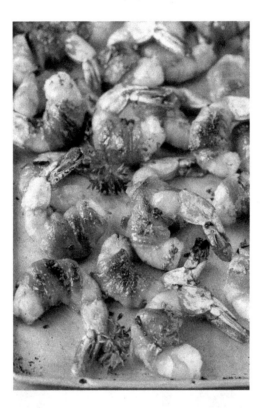

### Ingredients

- ½ cup freshly squeezed lemon juice
- ¼ cup EVOO
- ½ cup chopped fresh cilantro
- 1 garlic clove, minced
- 1 pound shrimp, peeled and deveined
- 1 (12-ounce) package nitrate-free bacon, strips halved widthwise

### Directions

1. Preheat the oven to 350°F. Line a baking sheet with parchment paper and set aside.
2. In a large bowl, whisk the lemon juice, EVOO, cilantro, and garlic.
3. Add the shrimp to the dressing. Gently mix to coat the shrimp evenly.
4. Wrap each shrimp in a piece of bacon and place on the prepared baking sheet.
5. Bake for 20 to 25 minutes until the bacon is nice and crispy.

Parsley & Garlic Scallops

Prep & Cooking time: 20 minutes
Serves: 4 to 6

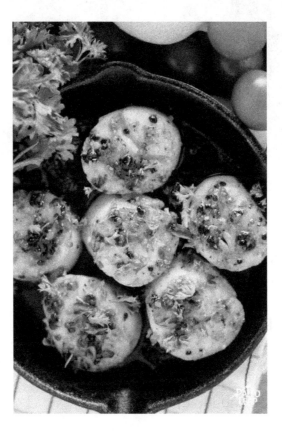

## Ingredients

- ⅓ cup EVOO
- 4 garlic cloves, minced
- 1½ pounds sea scallops
- 1 tablespoon paprika
- Juice of 2 lemons, plus zest from the lemons reserved for garnishing
- ½ cup minced fresh parsley, 2 tablespoons reserved for garnishing
- Sea salt
- Freshly ground black pepper

## Directions

1. In a large skillet over medium heat, heat the EVOO. Add the garlic and stir.
2. Add the scallops to the skillet and season with the paprika.
3. Add the lemon juice and parsley. Cook the scallops for 2 to 3 minutes per side to sear.
4. Serve the scallops warm, seasoned with sea salt and pepper, and garnished with the reserved lemon zest and parsley.

Salmon Burgers

Prep & Cooking time: 25 minutes
Serves: 4 to 6

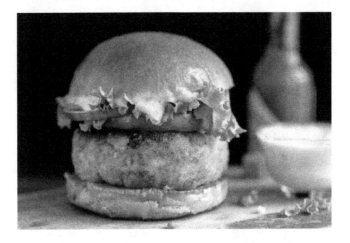

## Ingredients

- 1½ pounds salmon
- 2 large eggs
- 1 red onion, chopped
- ½ cup minced fresh dill
- 1 teaspoon red pepper flakes (optional)
- Sea salt
- Freshly ground black pepper
- 1 tablespoon EVOO
- 4 to 6 cooked sweet potatoes, cooled, peeled, and halved through the middle lengthwise (for buns)
- Sliced pickles, for serving (optional)

## Directions

1. In a large bowl, combine the salmon, eggs, red onion, dill, and red pepper flakes (if using). Gently stir to combine. Season with sea salt and black pepper. Form the mixture into 4 to 6 patties.
2. In a large skillet over medium-high heat, heat the EVOO.
3. Add the salmon patties (you may have to work in batches). Cook for about 5 minutes per side until nicely browned and crisp on the outside and cooked through.
4. Serve on a sweet potato "bun" with a pickle slice (if using) and other toppings as desired.


Salmon & Peaches

Prep & Cooking time: 30 minutes
Serves: 4 to 6

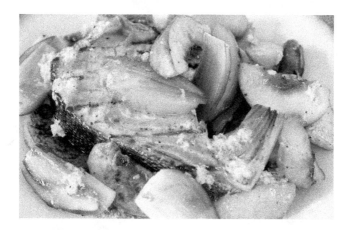

## Ingredients

- ½ cup EVOO, plus more for drizzling
- ½ cup finely chopped fresh cilantro
- 1 medium red onion, diced
- 2 tablespoons minced peeled fresh ginger
- Sea salt
- Freshly ground black pepper
- 4 to 6 (6-ounce) salmon fillets
- 4 cups sliced fresh peaches

## Directions

1. Preheat the oven to 350°F. Line a baking sheet with parchment paper and set it aside.
2. In a small bowl, whisk the EVOO, cilantro, red onion, and ginger. Season with sea salt and pepper. Whisk again to combine.
3. Place the salmon on the baking sheet and brush the cilantro dressing over it, giving it a nice coat.
4. Place the sliced peaches on top of and around the salmon. Drizzle the peaches with EVOO.
5. Bake the salmon and peaches for 20 to 25 minutes, or until the salmon are nice and crispy and the peaches are nicely browned.

*VARIATION TIP:* Use sliced fresh pineapple rings instead of the peaches for a more tropical flavor.


## Lemon-Garlic Shrimp & Tomatoes

Prep & Cooking time: 20 minutes
Serves: 4 to 6

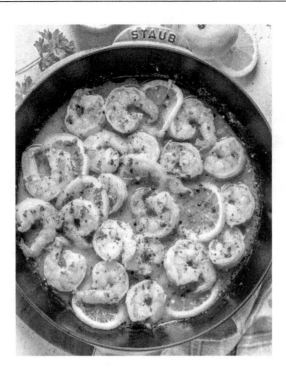

## Ingredients

- ½ cup ghee
- 1½ pounds shrimp, peeled and deveined
- 6 to 8 garlic cloves, minced
- 1 cup chopped fresh basil, 2 tablespoons reserved for garnishing
- 1 cup chopped fresh cilantro, 2 tablespoons reserved for garnishing
- 2 cups heirloom cherry tomatoes
- 2 lemons, halved

## Directions

1. In a sauté pan or large skillet over medium-high heat, heat the ghee. Add the shrimp. Cook for 2 to 5 minutes until it starts to turn pink.
2. Sprinkle the minced garlic over the shrimp. Add the basil and cilantro, and toss to combine. Sauté everything for a few minutes more until the shrimp is mostly cooked.
3. Add the cherry tomatoes. Sauté for 5 minutes more until the tomatoes start to pop. Transfer to serving dishes. Squeeze fresh lemon juice over everything. Garnish with the reserved basil and cilantro.

*MAKE IT EASIER TIP:* Buy shrimp that has already been peeled and deveined. It costs a bit more but will save you a ton of prep time.

### Easy Barbecue Chicken

Prep time: 1 hour 15 minutes
Serves: 4 to 6

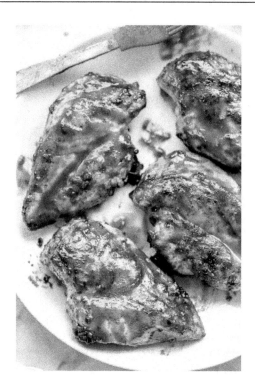

## Ingredients

- 2 cups Barbecue Sauce or store-bought sugar-free chemical-free barbecue sauce
- 3 tablespoons coconut aminos
- 1 teaspoon chili powder
- Sea salt
- Freshly ground black pepper
- 4 to 6 chicken legs

## Directions

1. Preheat the oven to 425°F. Line a baking sheet with parchment paper and set it aside.
2. In a small bowl, stir together the barbecue sauce, coconut aminos, and chili powder. Season with sea salt and pepper. Stir again to combine.
3. Using a pastry brush, coat each chicken leg with the sauce and then give each leg a second coat. Place the basted legs on the prepared baking sheet 1 inch apart.
4. Bake for 50 to 60 minutes until the chicken is nice and crispy and the juices run clear.

Variation tip: For a smoky flavor, cook this chicken on the grill. Preheat a grill to medium-high heat. Coat the chicken in the sauce mixture and place it on the grill. Cook for 20 to 30 minutes, basting occasionally with the remaining sauce mixture and turning halfway through cooking until cooked through.

Veggie & Chicken Bake

Prep & Cooking time: 1 hour 10 minutes
Serves: 4 to 6

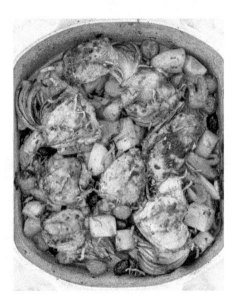

## Ingredients

- 1 cup coconut aminos
- 1½ pounds boneless skinless chicken breast, cubed
- 2 tablespoons chopped garlic
- Sea salt
- Freshly ground black pepper
- 2 cups broccoli florets
- 2 cups sliced green beans
- 1 medium red onion, diced

## Directions

1. Preheat the oven to 350°F.
2. Place the coconut aminos in a skillet and place the skillet over medium-high heat.
3. Add the chicken and garlic. Season with sea salt and pepper. Cook the chicken for 10 minutes, or until it's no longer pink in the middle.
4. Place half each of the broccoli, green beans, and red onion in a casserole dish in a single layer.
5. Add the chicken. Top the chicken with the remaining veggies.
6. Bake for 40 to 50 minutes until everything is nice and crispy.

Variation tip: Substitute other nonstarchy veggies you have on hand. Mushrooms, asparagus, bell peppers, and summer squash all work well here.


Coconut-Crusted Calamari

Prep & Cooking time: 20 minutes
Serves: 4 to 6

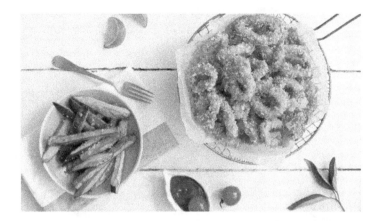

## Ingredients

- 1 cup ghee, melted
- 2 cups unsweetened shredded coconut
- 2 cups coconut flour
- 4 cups coconut oil
- 1⅓ pounds cleaned squid, cut into rings
- Flaky sea salt
- ¼ cup freshly squeezed lemon juice
- Cocktail sauce, for serving

## Directions

1. Place the melted ghee in a medium bowl. In another medium bowl, whisk the coconut and coconut flour.
2. In a deep skillet over medium heat, melt the coconut oil, letting it get hot. You'll know when the oil is ready when it begins to bubble slightly.
3. Dip a piece of calamari into the ghee and dip it into the coconut mixture, coating the calamari well. Repeat to coat all the calamari.
4. Using a slotted spoon, carefully place several pieces of calamari into the hot oil, but be careful not to crowd the pan. Cook for 30 seconds to 1 minute until browned. Using a slotted spoon, transfer to paper towels to drain. Repeat until all the calamari is cooked.

5. Sprinkle the calamari with sea salt, drizzle with lemon juice, and serve with the cocktail sauce for dipping.

*PRO TIP:* To minimize the mess when deep-frying, use a high-sided pot, such as a Dutch oven. A cast-iron Dutch oven (either enameled or uncoated) makes a great deep-frying pot because it conducts heat well and contains splatters.


Chicken Fajita Bowls

Prep & Cooking time: 20 minutes
Serves: 4 to 6

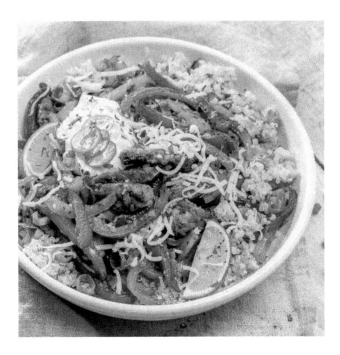

## Ingredients

- 1 tablespoon coconut oil
- 2 boneless skinless chicken breasts, cubed
- 1 medium red onion, chopped
- 2 bell peppers, any color or a mix, cored and sliced
- 2 cups fresh corn kernels
- 1 head purple cauliflower, cut into florets
- Sea salt
- Freshly ground black pepper
- Full-fat coconut cream, for serving (optional)

## Directions

1. In a skillet over medium-high heat, heat the coconut oil.
2. Add the chicken to the skillet, followed by the red onion. Reduce the heat to medium and sauté until the chicken begins to brown, about 5 minutes.
3. Add the bell peppers, corn, and purple cauliflower. Sauté for 10 minutes until everything is cooked thoroughly. Season with sea salt and pepper. Serve topped with coconut cream (if using).

# Chapter 4: Desserts

Homemade Caramel-Dipped Apples

Serves 4
Prep & Cooking time: 25 minutes

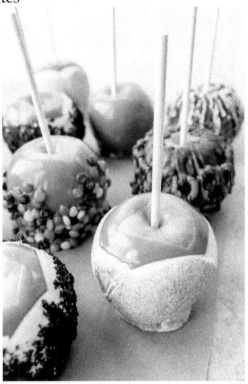

## Ingredients
- Equipment: 4 wooden skewers
- 4 Pink Lady, Honeycrisp, Fuji, or Granny Smith apples
- Cooking spray
- ½ cup Homemade Caramel Sauce
- ½ cup unsalted peanuts, chopped

## Directions
1. Remove the stems of the apples, and push a wooden skewer into the bottom of each apple, about three-quarters of the way through.
2. Line a baking sheet with parchment paper and coat with cooking spray.
3. Warm the caramel sauce in a microwave-safe bowl for 1 minute, stirring frequently.
4. Quickly roll each apple in the caramel sauce. Use a spoon to cover the apple with the sauce.
5. Roll or dip the caramel apples in the chopped nuts, then place them on the prepared baking sheet. Refrigerate until the caramel hardens, about 15 minutes.

Per serving: Calories: 311; Total fat: 16g; Saturated fat: 6g; Protein: 5g; Carbohydrates: 40g; Fiber: 6g; Sodium: 64mg

## Coconut-Date Pudding

Serves 4
Prep & Cooking time: 3 hours 20 minutes

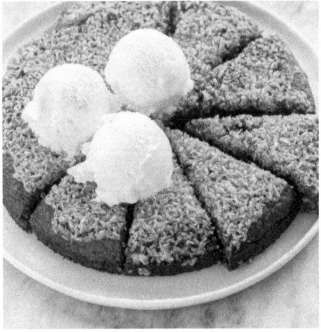

### Ingredients
- Equipment: 4 (8-ounce) ramekins
- 3 cups unsweetened coconut milk, divided
- 1½ cups pitted Medjool dates, chopped
- 4 tablespoons (¼ cup) chopped walnuts
- 3 tablespoons water
- 1 teaspoon gelatin
- 1 teaspoon ground cinnamon

### Directions
1. In a medium saucepan, bring 1 cup of coconut milk and the dates to a boil. Reduce heat to medium-low, and continue cooking, stirring often, until the liquid evaporates, about 5 minutes.
2. Divide the dates between the 4 ramekins, pressing them into the bottom. Top the dates in each ramekin with 1 tablespoon of walnuts.
3. Add the remaining 2 cups of coconut milk to the saucepan, and heat over medium heat.
4. In a small bowl, whisk the water and gelatin, then add to the saucepan. Bring to a boil, reduce heat to medium, and whisk for about 5 minutes, until the gelatin is incorporated. Add the cinnamon, stirring to blend. Remove from heat and allow to slightly cool.
5. Pour the coconut mixture evenly between the 4 ramekins. Loosely cover with plastic wrap, and refrigerate the puddings to set for at least 3 hours or up to overnight.

Per serving: Calories: 334; Total fat: 10g; Saturated fat: 9g; Protein: 5g; Carbohydrates: 67g; Fiber: 8g; Sodium: 46mg

### Strawberry Compote in Red Wine Syrup

Serves 4
Prep & Cooking time: 30 minutes

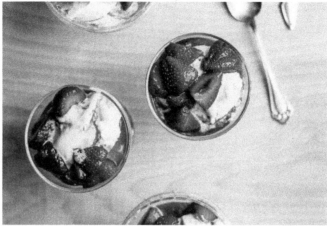

## Ingredients
- 1 cup red wine
- ⅓ cup granulated sugar
- 1 teaspoon vanilla extract
- ½ teaspoon ground cinnamon
- 4 cups strawberries, hulled and sliced

## Directions
1. In a medium saucepan, bring the wine, sugar, vanilla, and cinnamon to a boil. Reduce heat and simmer until the liquid is reduced by half, about 20 minutes.
2. Place 1 cup of berries into each of 4 cups. Drizzle with 2 tablespoons of the red wine syrup.
3. Serve warm or chill in the refrigerator before serving.

Per serving: Calories: 119; Total fat: 0g; Saturated fat: 0g; Protein: 1g; Carbohydrates: 28g; Fiber: 3g; Sodium: 2mg


### Milk Chocolate Peanut Butter Cups

Serves 12
Prep & Cooking time: 1 hour 25 minutes

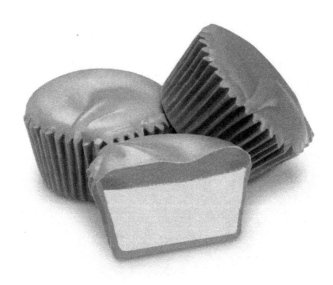

## Ingredients

- Cooking spray
- 12 ounces milk chocolate, broken into pieces
- 2 tablespoons coconut oil
- 12 teaspoons natural creamy peanut butter
- ⅛ teaspoon sea salt

## Directions

1. Spray 12 mini-muffin liners with cooking spray, then place in an 8-by-8 dish.
2. In a small saucepan, bring a cup of water to a boil, then reduce heat to a simmer. Fit a heat-proof medium bowl on top of the saucepan to make a double boiler. Add the chocolate and coconut oil to the bowl, stirring gently with a wooden spoon until smooth, about 5 minutes.
3. Fill one-third of each muffin liner with melted chocolate, then 1 teaspoon of peanut butter, and top with melted chocolate.
4. Transfer the dish to the refrigerator and allow to sit for at least 1 hour.

Per serving: Calories: 194; Total fat: 12g; Saturated fat: 7g; Protein: 3g; Carbohydrates: 21g; Fiber: 1g; Sodium: 66mg


Chocolate-Dipped Citrus Fruit

Serves 10
Prep & Cooking time: 35 minutes

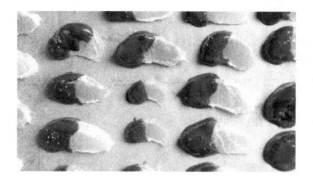

## Ingredients

- 4 ounces 60% dark chocolate, broken into pieces
- 1 tablespoon coconut oil
- 3 clementines, peeled and segmented
- 1 navel orange, peeled and segmented
- 3 mandarin oranges, peeled and segmented

## Directions

1. Line a baking sheet with parchment paper.
2. In a small saucepan, bring about a cup of water to a boil, then reduce heat to a simmer. Place a heat-proof medium bowl on top of the saucepan to make a double boiler. Add the chocolate and coconut oil, and stir gently with a wooden spoon until the mixture is smooth about 5 minutes.
3. One at a time, dip the tip of each citrus segment into the melted chocolate, and place onto the prepared baking sheet, leaving about ½ inch between pieces.
4. Place in the refrigerator to set, about 15 minutes.

Per serving: Calories: 92; Total fat: 5g; Saturated fat: 3g; Protein 1g; Carbohydrates: 11g; Fiber: 2g; Sodium: 1mg

## Banana-Cinnamon "Ice Cream"

Serves 4
Prep & Cooking time: 10 minutes

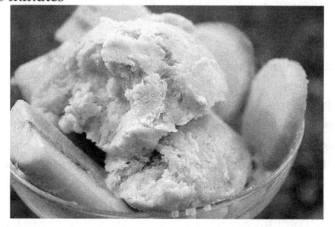

## Ingredients

- 4 medium frozen bananas, cut into 2-inch chunks
- ¼ cup 100% maple syrup
- 1 teaspoon ground cinnamon

## Directions

1. Allow the frozen banana chunks to rest at room temperature for 5 minutes, then place in a food processor or blender.
2. Add the maple syrup and cinnamon, and purée until well combined.
3. Serve immediately, or store in a freezer-safe container in the freezer until later.

Per serving: Calories: 159; Total fat: 0g; Saturated fat: 0g; Protein: 1g; Carbohydrates: 41 g; Fiber: 3g; Sodium: 4mg

Berry Yogurt Trifle

Serves 8
Prep & Cooking time: 45 minutes

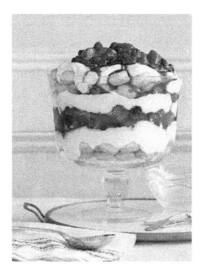

## Ingredients

- 2 cups nonfat vanilla Greek yogurt
- 2 tablespoons honey
- 1 (10-ounce) store-bought angel food cake, cut into 1-inch cubes
- 1½ cups strawberries, hulled and halved
- 1½ cups blueberries
- 1 cup Vanilla-Infused Whipped Cream

## Directions

1. In a small bowl, mix the yogurt and honey.
2. In a large bowl or trifle dish, distribute half of the angel food cake in an even layer. Top the cake with 1 cup of the yogurt mixture, using a spatula to evenly coat. Top with half of the strawberries and blueberries. Repeat to make a second layer, then top with the whipped cream.
3. Cover and refrigerate to set, about 30 minutes.

Per serving: Calories: 243; Total fat 6g; Saturated fat: 4g; Protein: 8g; Carbohydrates: 41 g; Fiber: 2g; Sodium: 291 mg

Honey-Peach Ice Pops

Serves 6
Prep & Cooking time: 4 hours 10 minutes

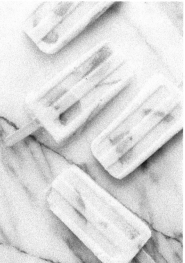

## Ingredients
- Equipment: 6 ice pop molds
- 1¼ cups diced fresh or thawed frozen peaches
- 1 cup nonfat vanilla Greek yogurt
- 2 tablespoons 100% maple syrup
- ¼ cup 2% fat milk
- 2 teaspoons freshly squeezed lemon juice
- ½ teaspoon ground cinnamon

## Directions
1. In a blender, add the peaches, yogurt, syrup, milk, lemon juice, and cinnamon, and blend until smooth.
2. Using a ¼-cup scoop, pour the purée into the ice pop molds, and top each with a stick.
3. Freeze until set, at least 4 hours.

Per serving: Calories: 63; Total fat: 0g; Saturated fat: 0g; Protein: 3g; Carbohydrates: 12g; Fiber: 1g; Sodium: 18mg


Ellena's Peanut Butter Cookies

Makes 14 cookies
Prep & Cooking time: 35 minutes

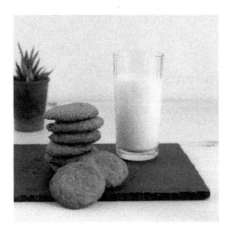

## Ingredients
- Cooking spray
- 1 cup packed light brown sugar
- 1 large egg
- 1 teaspoon vanilla extract
- 1 cup natural creamy peanut butter
- ⅛ teaspoon salt

## Directions
1. Preheat the oven to 350°F. Coat a baking sheet with cooking spray.
2. In a medium bowl, whisk together the brown sugar, egg, and vanilla.
3. Add the peanut butter and salt, mixing well to combine.
4. Scoop out 1 teaspoon of the batter, and use clean hands to roll into a ball. Place on the prepared baking sheet, pressing down to flatten. Repeat with the remaining batter, leaving ½ inch between cookies.
5. Bake on the center rack in the oven for 18 to 20 minutes, until the cookies are golden brown.
6. Remove from the oven and allow the cookies to cool for 5 minutes. Transfer the cookies to a wire rack to finish cooling for at least 10 minutes before serving.

Per serving: Calories: 173; Total fat: 9g; Saturated fat: 2g; Protein: 4g; Carbohydrates: 20g; Fiber: 1g; Sodium: 118mg


Flourless Double-Chocolate Chip Cookies

Makes 15 cookies
Prep & Cooking time: 30 minutes

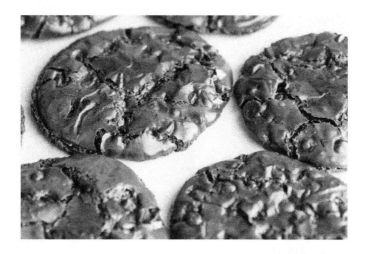

## Ingredients

- Cooking spray
- 1 cup creamy almond butter
- 6 tablespoons honey
- 1 tablespoon unsweetened cocoa powder
- 2 large eggs
- ⅓ teaspoon salt
- ⅓ cup semisweet chocolate chips

## Directions

1. Preheat the oven to 350°F. Coat a baking sheet with cooking spray.
2. In a blender, add the almond butter, honey, cocoa powder, eggs, and salt, and blend until smooth. Fold in the chocolate chips.
3. Scoop out 1 teaspoon of batter, and use clean hands to form into a ball. Place on the prepared baking sheet, pressing to flatten into a disc. Repeat with the remaining batter, leaving 1 inch between cookies.
4. Bake on the center rack in the oven for 12 to 15 minutes, until the cookies are golden brown.
5. Remove from the oven and allow the cookies to cool for 5 minutes. Transfer to a wire rack to finish cooling for at least 10 minutes before serving.

Per serving: Calories: 159; Total fat: 11g; Saturated fat: 1g; Protein: 5g; Carbohydrates: 13g; Fiber: 2g; Sodium: 88mg


Almond Macaroons

Makes 16 macaroons
Prep & Cooking time: 30 minutes

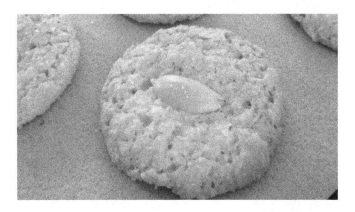

## Ingredients

- 1 (7-ounce) package unsweetened coconut flakes
- ⅔ cup sweetened condensed milk
- ⅓ cup raw almonds, finely chopped
- ¼ cup honey
- 1 teaspoon almond extract
- 3 egg whites

## Directions

1. Preheat the oven to 350°F. Line a baking sheet with parchment paper.
2. In a medium bowl, add the coconut, milk, almonds, honey, and almond extract, and stir to combine.
3. In another medium bowl, add the egg whites. Using an electric hand mixer, beat the egg whites until soft peaks form.
4. Gently fold the beaten egg whites into the coconut mixture.
5. Spoon out 1 heaping tablespoon of the mixture. Use clean hands to roll into a ball and place on the prepared baking sheet. Continue with the remainder of the batter, leaving about 1 inch between macaroons.
6. Bake for 12 to 15 minutes, until the macaroons are lightly browned.

Per serving: Calories: 164; Total fat: 11g; Saturated fat: 8g; Protein: 3g; Carbohydrates: 16g; Fiber: 2g; Sodium: 30mg

Banana-Oat Walnut Loaf

Serves 8
Prep & Cooking time: 40 minutes

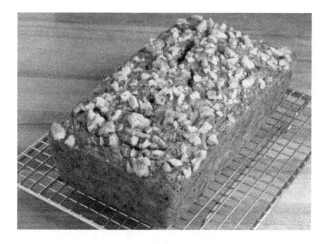

## Ingredients

- Cooking spray
- 2 cups gluten-free rolled oats, plus 2 tablespoons
- 3 ripe bananas, mashed
- 2 large eggs, lightly beaten
- ½ cup honey
- 1 teaspoon baking soda
- ½ cup raw walnuts, chopped

## Directions

1. Preheat the oven to 350°F. Coat an 8-inch loaf pan with cooking spray.
2. In a medium bowl, mix 2 cups of oats and the mashed bananas, beaten eggs, honey, and baking soda. Gently fold in the walnuts.
3. Pour the mixture into the prepared pan, spreading in an even layer with a spatula. Sprinkle the remaining 2 tablespoons of oats on top of the batter.
4. Bake for about 25 minutes, until the top is golden brown and a toothpick inserted into the center comes out clean. Remove from the oven and allow to cool for 10 minutes. Transfer the bread to a wire rack and let cool for 10 to 15 more minutes, then cut into 1-inch slices.
5. To freeze, place each slice in a resealable plastic bag or wrap them individually in plastic wrap and store the slices in the freezer for up to 2 months. To defrost, refrigerate overnight. The loaf can be eaten at room temperature, warmed in a toaster oven, or reheated in the microwave on high for 20 to 30 seconds. Allow the slices to cool for 2 minutes after reheating in the microwave before eating.

Per serving: Calories: 205; Total fat: 6g; Saturated fat: 1g; Protein: 4g; Carbohydrates: 36g; Fiber: 3g; Sodium: 122mg

## Quick Chocolate Cake

Serves 8
Prep & Cooking time: 50 minutes

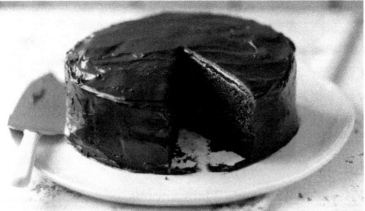

### Ingredients
- Cooking spray
- 4 ounces semisweet chocolate, broken into pieces
- 6 tablespoons (¾ stick) unsalted butter, cut into pieces
- ¾ cup granulated sugar
- 3 large eggs
- 1 cup unbleached all-purpose flour

### Directions
1. Preheat the oven to 425°F. Coat an 8-inch round cake pan with cooking spray.
2. In a microwave-safe bowl, add the chocolate and butter on high at 30-second intervals, stirring between each interval, until smooth, about 2 minutes.
3. Using an electric mixer, mix the sugar and eggs until the mixture thickens. Add the flour and continue to mix until combined. Add the chocolate mixture, and mix to incorporate.
4. Pour the batter into the prepared cake pan, and bake for 22 to 25 minutes, until a toothpick inserted into the cake comes out clean.
5. Remove from the oven and allow to cool for at least 15 minutes. Cut into 8 pieces and serve.

Per serving: Calories: 303; Total fat: 15g; Saturated fat: 9g; Protein: 5g; Carbohydrates: 39g; Fiber: 1g; Sodium: 28mg

## Applelicious Apple Crisp

Serves 6
Prep & Cooking time: 55 minutes

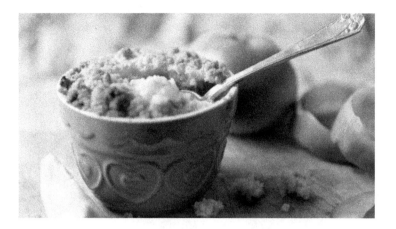

## Ingredients
FOR THE FILLING
- Cooking spray
- 6 medium apples (like Empire, Honey crisp, Pink Lady), cored and thinly sliced
- 2 tablespoons honey

FOR THE TOPPING
- ¾ cup old-fashioned oats
- ¾ cup whole-wheat pastry flour
- ⅓ cup light brown sugar
- 3 tablespoons unsalted butter, at room temperature, cut into pieces
- 3 tablespoons water

## Directions
1. Preheat the oven to 350°F. Coat an 8-by-8-inch baking dish with cooking spray.
2. Place the apples in a medium bowl. Add the honey and toss to coat. Transfer to the prepared baking dish.
3. To make the topping, in a blender, add the oats, flour, brown sugar, butter, and water, and blend until smooth.
4. Use clean fingers to crumble the topping over the apples.
5. Place the baking dish in the middle rack of the oven, and bake for 40 minutes, until the topping is browned and the apples are cooked through.
6. Remove from the oven and allow to cool for at least 10 minutes. Using a spoon, divide the crisp into six portions and serve.

Per serving: Calories: 268; Total fat: 7g; Saturated fat: 4g; Protein: 3g; Carbohydrates: 51 g; Fiber: 6g; Sodium: 2mg


Slow Cooker Poached Pears with Pomegranate Sauce

Serves 4
Prep & Cooking time: 1 hour 45 minutes

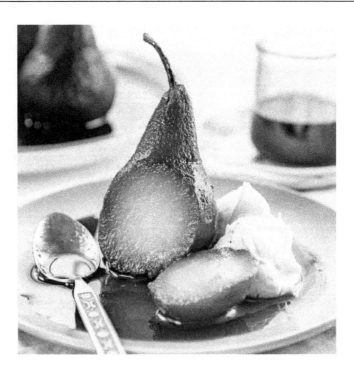

## Ingredients

- 4 pears, peeled, halved, and cored
- 1½ cups 100% pomegranate juice
- 3 tablespoons flavored vodka (optional)
- 2 tablespoons 100% maple syrup
- ½ teaspoon ground cinnamon

## Directions

1. Place the pears, cut-side down, in the slow cooker.
2. In a small bowl, whisk together the pomegranate juice, vodka (if using), syrup, and cinnamon, and pour over the pears.
3. Cover and cook on low until the pear is fork-soft, about 90 minutes.

Per serving: Calories: 181; Total fat: 1g; Saturated fat: 0g; Protein: 1g; Carbohydrates: 46g; Fiber: 6g; Sodium: 11mg

# Measurement conversion table

## VOLUME EQUIVALENTS (LIQUID)

| US STANDARD | US STANDARD (OUNCES) | METRIC (APPROXIMATE) |
| --- | --- | --- |
| 2 tablespoons | 1 fl. oz. | 30 mL |
| ¼ cup | 2 fl. oz. | 60 mL |
| ½ cup | 4 fl. oz. | 120 mL |
| 1 cup | 8 fl. oz. | 240 mL |
| 1½ cups | 12 fl. oz. | 355 mL |
| 2 cups or 1 pint | 16 fl. oz. | 475 mL |
| 4 cups or 1 quart | 32 fl. oz. | 1 L |
| 1 gallon | 128 fl. oz. | 4 L |

## OVEN TEMPERATURES

| FAHRENHEIT | CELSIUS (APPROXIMATE) |
| --- | --- |
| 250°F | 120°C |
| 300°F | 150°C |
| 325°F | 165°C |
| 350°F | 180°C |
| 375°F | 190°C |
| 400°F | 200°C |
| 425°F | 220°C |
| 450°F | 230°C |

## VOLUME EQUIVALENTS (DRY)

| US STANDARD | METRIC (APPROXIMATE) |
| --- | --- |
| ⅛ teaspoon | 0.5 mL |
| ¼ teaspoon | 1 mL |
| ½ teaspoon | 2 mL |
| ¾ teaspoon | 4 mL |
| 1 teaspoon | 5 mL |
| 1 tablespoon | 15 mL |
| ¼ cup | 59 mL |
| ⅓ cup | 79 mL |
| ½ cup | 118 mL |
| ⅔ cup | 156 mL |
| ¾ cup | 177 mL |
| 1 cup | 235 mL |
| 2 cups or 1 pint | 475 mL |
| 3 cups | 700 mL |
| 4 cups or 1 quart | 1 L |

## WEIGHT EQUIVALENTS

| US STANDARD | METRIC (APPROXIMATE) |
| --- | --- |
| ½ ounce | 15 g |
| 1 ounce | 30 g |
| 2 ounces | 60 g |
| 4 ounces | 115 g |

| 8 ounces | 225 g |
|---|---|
| 12 ounces | 340 g |
| 16 ounces or 1 pound | 455 g |

# Quick Prep Paleo

Whole-Food Meals with 5 to 15 Minutes of Hand-On-

Time for Smart People on a Budget

Chef John Tank

# Table of Contents

# Introduction

This book is for fun loving, taste focused people who love to cook and eat yummy Paleo diets made using slow cooker. You can get better understandings about the Paleo slow cooker cuisine, as well as its health benefits on the Introduction folio. This book comprises the collection of recipes for every meal of the day and healthy lives. First of all, in chapter – 1 you find basic guide about the Paleo diet and cooking by using slow cooker. Next, in chapter – 2 are the light and delicious appetizer recipes which are your starter point to paleo cuisine. In chapter – 3, you will find luscious breakfast recipes. Then, in chapter - 4, you will find the healthy and delicious lunch recipes. Then comes the fiery dinner recipes which are grouped in chapter - 5. Last but not the least; indulge your sweet tooth without even breaking the rules! Enjoy the collection of delicious & nutritious slow cooked desserts & snacks recipes while getting into your new habits in chapter - 6. These delicious and healthy recipes will definitely provides you the best nutritious and health benefits that your bodies needs.

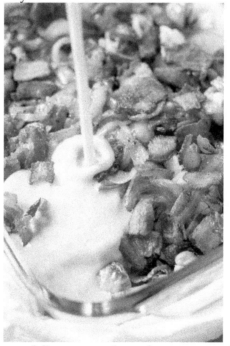

The human diet is a diverse range of flavors and preferences, and has evolved enormously with time. 10,000 years ago cavemen used to hunt for food and devour vegetables and fruits that grew on land. They fished from the sea and hunted wild beasts for their meat. This has been referred to as the Paleolilith era that advocated an organic diet that sufficed to say, was regarded as the diet for optimum health by scientists and doctors. Since, the emergence of agriculture, various toxins and additives have made their way into out diet and have started a chain reaction of several different medical problems like immune system disorders, celiac diseases, and other autoimmune diseases that overtime can cripple human health.

The purpose of this book is not just to take a look at the Paleo diet as a serious health upgrade diet, but it is also to take a peek into the world of Paleo desserts because most people wrongly assume that being on a Paleo diet means you can't have desserts. Let's face it we don't know what desserts were available to the cavemen in their time and it could be really hard to grasp that once you're on a Paleo diet you won't enjoy a cupcake again.

This is the very point with which most scientists and nutrition experts have a beef about with the Paleo diet. They counteract Paleo diet principles with damning views over how due to the vast evolution of human diet, reverting back to a caveman's diet is not something that is altogether doable. Cavemen never had our technology, or ability to cultivate grains and wheat. In the opinion of modern nutritionists, the caveman diet is as obsolete as a typewriter with the explosion of new technology. While, they are right to establish that the human tastes and flavors have expanded to new levels that were beyond the scope of cavemen, the Paleo diet isn't really about being a caveman, it's about adapting our diet to meet the organic goodness that sheltered human beings 12000 years ago, and nurtured their bodies with nutrition value that is quite frankly lacking in processed foods and produce of today.

No, Paleo does not mean you go cold turkey on desserts. In fact, the Paleo diet encourages desserts made of organic and fresh products that don't just serve as empty calories, or make you slave to overeating with their high fructose sugar content. Another modern-day sucrose conversion that is addictive and present in most foods and drinks, drinks especially, due to its solubility level.

Let's take a look at what the Paleo diet is and what it has to offer.

# What Is Paleo

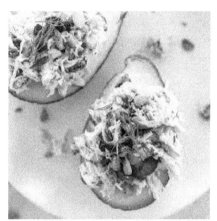

The Paleo diet is one of the most unquestionably interesting diet concepts that have racked up the points in the last few decades. Everyone from celebrities to the general public are adopting it left, right, and center, as the secret of their healthy glow. Health diets and fad diets generally tell you to skimp on desserts, or just altogether forego the bite of a heavenly cream doughnut, but you would be happy to learn that the Paleo diet is one such diet that does not dissuade you from eating those comfort goodies.

The Paleo Diet is the planet's most healthy diet generally based on consuming delightful, up to date foods which have nutritive approach in order that it works rather well body genetics to help remain lean, powerful and energized. The name comes from Paleolithic age, or the Stone Age, when the forbears were hunters and gatherers of natural foods.

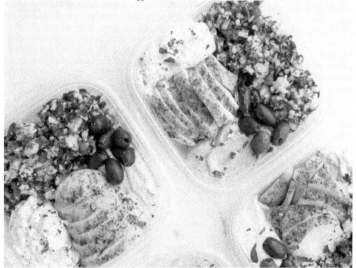

It in fact, encourages your sweet tooth, but with some adaptive changes that allow for organic ingredients to make up decadent treats that leave your mouth watering for more.

There are several reasons you may have decided to go for Paleo as a lifestyle change, but the need for a dessert treat every now and then remains constant.

So, what is this book about?

This Paleo dessert cookbook is especially dedicated for people who love to celebrate St. Valentine's day and who love to enjoy eating scrumptious desserts without having to feel guilty about it and without having to sacrifice their love for
some sweet treats and desserts.

The healthy desserts & gluten paleo baking book will tell you why Paleo is the craze now and why you should be enjoying the Paleo lifestyle, too!

This grain free Paleo vegan sweets book for the Holidays will also tell you ways in which the Paleo diet will change your lifestyle for the better and turn guilt into guilt free pleasures

This Paleo cupcake and frosting recipes book will also tell you what ingredients to have in your kitchen as a staple for paleo dessert pleasures during the Holidays

This Valentines Day recipes book will give you 33 scrumptious Paleo desserts (Paleo Gluten Free & Grain Free Muffin Recipes, Paleo Cupcake And Frosting Recipes, Paleo Vegan Sweets & Paleo Smoothies) that you probably desire right now.

Inside the Paleo Holiday recipes book you will learn how to make these easy Paleo desserts in a quick & no fail fashion and even if you are a busy mom or a busy person who works a lot. You can do this because you will find some easy and quick fix 3 Minute Paleo Holiday recipes, too!

Based on the knowledge of this paleo dessert book you will be empowered and enabled to discover and explore more and more Paleo dessert applications by yourself and this is where the fun begins

You will absolutely learn how to turn guilt into guilt free pleasures by pure will power and indulge your partner and loved one with these scrumptious & healthy Holiday treats

Ultimately, you will be living some intensive and pleasurable Paleo dessert moments free from guilt and this is when you finally are able to live the paleo lifestyle beyond the Holidays because in the end you do not really want to give up eating these delicious desserts, but learn how to integrate them into the reality of your life while becoming healthier and fitter every day!

## Why Paleo Desserts Work

You must be wondering why would you want to take a look at Paleo as a serious diet change to improve your lifestyle and health?

There is no shortage of medical journals and newspaper articles, internet bites, and TV infomercials that tell us what is good for the body, what is good for your heart, and what processed food substance will lower your bodies cholesterol. Earlier men and women had longer lives and lesser issues with their health because of natural and organic diets. This in itself should make you question what are you putting in your bodies these days and what are you feeding your children alike? You may find yourself easily tired at say, age 35, while your father at that age was a tough sport about marathoning through work hours, juggling family, and social activities alike. This is proof that even with evolved diets, eating organic food and eating less processed junk did their bodies actual good.

Now let's enter the Paleo world. As with any other diets, one would be cautious about its overall effect on our body and mind. Scientific studies, while not a hundred percent accurate, but still, many studies have shown that Paleolilith men/women suffered from none of the hundreds of modern diseases that have been on the rise like an epidemic after the evolution of our diet, and the

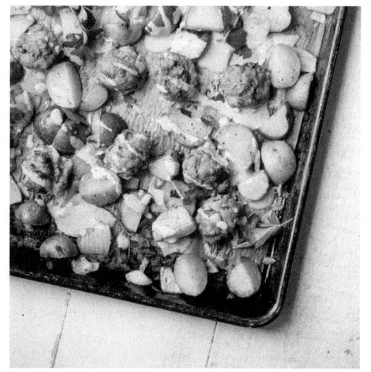

introductions of agricultural additives and processed food additives that have done the opposite of nurturing our bodies.

But as they all say the proof is in the pudding. Most people who have adapted this lifestyle have nothing but good things to say about this diet. Most importantly, this diet has helped many severely affected patients of different autoimmune diseases achieve restoration of their health almost immediately.

Most of us only hear about gluten in products and how it affects 'some' people badly. If you've heard about gluten free products several times, and don't know why gluten is a common enemy affecting 1 in 100 cases then, let' talk about gluten.

Gluten is a protein present in all wheat based products and all its cross breeds like rye and barley as well. Today most processed food items apart from wheat products themselves also contain gluten, and it seems that more than some people are badly affecting by the presence of this protein in their foods.

Gluten has been linked to most autoimmune diseases, diarrhea, leaky gut syndrome, intestinal damage, and fatigue to name just a few. The worst part is that most of us don't even know that we may be suffering from any gluten allergies. Many cases of celiac disease remain undiagnosed because sometimes the symptoms are subtle and grow over time, or just don't affect us as severely as it does to some people with diagnosed cases of celiac disease.

Paleo is not just a gluten free diet, it is also a low carb and high fat that encourages the use of some nutritional fat that helps to create energy in a human body. Due to obvious myths that have been fed to us over time through commercials, articles, and scientists we feel afraid of the very mention of 'FAT' in our diet and disregard a high fat diet as complete misnomer.

Fat is not always bad, and carbohydrates only provide energy to that gets burned away immediately. Fats are another macronutrient that give your body the energy to get through the day. Proof of this is the cavemen themselves. They existed on high fat diets that allowed them energy and alertness to hunt and gather for themselves. That can be an intense workout by modern day standards. Out complicated routines of this day is nothing short of intense effort and exertion. A high fat diet will assist in enriching your lifestyle in many ways.

Another issue in our general diet is how our non-Paleo lifestyle affects your blood sugar level and how quickly the blood glucose level rises. All foods have varying glycemic levels (the rate at how quickly your blood sugar level rises with a food) and some make your blood sugar levels increase).

If it's still hard to get a handle on why Paleo should be your diet then let's take a look at the fat free craze that has been on the roll for the last few decades. Fats and saturated fats are both touted as 'evils' that encourage cholesterol and bad heart health, but this is a one-sided story. Let's not delve into heavy medical and cellular jargon for it. Keeping it simple, saturated fats aren't all bad fats. Yes, there are good saturated fats, as well as bad saturated fats. The good fats contribute to good heart health, and don't encourage buildup of harmful triglycerides in arteries (what we call clogged arteries are the results of harmful triglycerides build up in our arteries). The macronutrients encouraged in Paleo are all sources of good saturated fats that are productive in increasing heart health and vitality.

Coming to the issue of losing weight with this diet, weight loss can be a seriously frustrating battle if your diet is the one that is hindering your success. Paleo is also know to help slim down those of us who have tried other diets and not found themselves close to shedding those annoying pounds. The low carb, high fat diet that Paleo encourages is also high in its protein quotient. A filling part of the equation that helps keep the individual satiated for longer, and revert to processed foods less. Once you cut out sugars, high carbs, and gluten out of your diet, you are bound to start dropping pounds. The high protein content also encourages more muscle development and promotes quicker fat burning.

Many organic ingredients in the Paleo diet encourage satiation of appetite and fat burning.

Based on this knowledge we can now move on to look at Paleo from the perspective of being a lifestyle choice that you can make for your own life.

## How Paleo Can Change Your Life: The Paleo Lifestyle

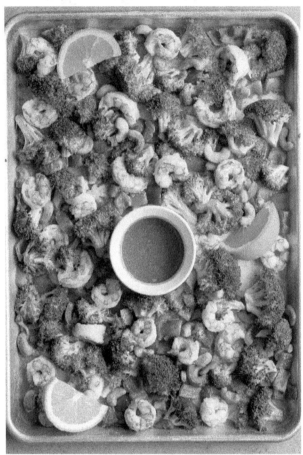

The Paleo diet has been called many things, and chief among them is the title of the caveman diet. A name that unwittingly turn some people off right away when they start imagining a bunch of drooling, hulking individuals beating their chests and running through the wild chasing wild beasts. That can be a disconcerting image, but Paleo is known as an all organic diet, and it is also touted as the low carb and high fat diet that can cleanse the body of toxins and additives of the modern processed foods epidemic.

Obesity, heart diseases, and food allergies (like gluten intolerance, celiac disease, diabetes, and other autoimmune disorders) have been on the rise for the last few decades. What hasn't eased these number in the last few years is the rising number of additives, like high fructose corn syrup, sodium, and 'bad' saturated fats in commercially processed cooking oils, and gluten in grains, wheat and all its byproducts.

We can't put an end to the production of these un-organic foods, but we can protect ourselves from further invasion of harmful diseases that may eventually cripple our body because of the empty calories they represent and their zero-nutritional value. Even fortified processed foods that claim to have Vitamins and minerals to make them look more appealing can be deceiving because of the really low percentage of the nutrients present in the foods. And even then, you may not be able to absorb those nutrients because of the presence of proteins that can inhibit our body's nutrient absorption by binding themselves to the nutrients and not letting them enter your blood stream.

Let's spell out what the Paleo diet is all about so that there is not confusion about what is shunned in the diet and how you can integrate the Paleo way of eating into your own lifestyle.

Before we do this, however, we must first clarify what ingredients to avoid with the Paleo lifestyle.

## Avoid list of Paleo Ingredients

1. Grains: Avoid all grains like rice, barley, wheat, rye, quinoa, millet, corn, amaranth, oats, etc. as all of these contain gluten in some degree.

2. Starchy vegetables: This means white potatoes. The high starch and high sugar content is not on recommended list in the Paleo diet.

3. Sugar: Eliminate sugar from your diet and stick to raw honey and Paleo substitutes such as unsweetened maple syrup (grade B) that avoid raising blood sugar levels exponentially.

4. Industrial and seed oils: Avoid vegetable and seed oils like peanut oils, sunflower, canola etc. because they are higher in 'bad' saturated fats, require more processing to become edible and easily go rancid, which creates health issues. Try oils like olive, coconut oil, ghee, and pure grass fed butter.

5. Legumes: all kinds of beans whether they be peas, mung beans, broad beans, garbanzo beans, lima beans, and/or peanuts. They have always been touted as healthy proteins, but are also high in carbohydrates and increase insulin release in your body.

6. Dairy: Another food source that increases insulin levels in human beings and can contain additives, antibiotics, and growth hormones that can all be harmful to your health.

7. Sodium: Use less sodium as it is known to cause bloating, water retention and harmful to human body in higher quantities. Limit your sodium consumption to 1000mg a day. Most processed foods contain sodium (canned beans, pre-made foods, deli meats, etc.) Try using sea salt instead it's a healthier Paleo option.

Paleo benefits

With this avoid list you must be thinking, how is avoiding any of this stuff make Paleo a good diet to be on? What are its benefits? After all if I'm giving up my pizza dough, I need to know it's got to be for some worthwhile reason. No way is any diet worth giving a try if you're going to be off the conventional pizza's made of gluten flour and fizzy drinks that are full of high fructose corn syrup.

Let's talk about some Paleo benefits that are sure to peak your interest.

Say goodbye to being 'hangry'. This is a combination of being both hungry and angry. Being on a high fat and low carbohydrate diet helps you stay satiated for longer. Some people experience rapid drop in their blood sugar,
which is followed by hunger and irritability. This is called hypoglycemia, but the Paleo diet will help with satiety and you will find yourself eating less than with other diets.

Experience sustained weight loss. Because of Paleo's food principles, you are consuming natural, organic, process free foods that help in controlling your weight. Processed carbs, sugar, and excess sodium are chief causes of weight gain. In a Paleo diet, once you get rid of foods that are discouraged by Paleo, you will notice a dramatic improvement in your weight and your ability to sustain that weight loss. Many studies have proved that things like high fructose corn syrup (a sweetener present in many processed food items) can be addictive. The HFCS is serving as empty calories itself, and your digestive system digests fructose in a different way from sucrose, but this is not the only cause of weight gain. HFCS is known to be addictive and when you drink one too many cans of some fizzy drink, you are bound to put on pounds.

No more bloating and being gassy all the time. You may have noticed that as you get older, eating certain foods causes your body to bloat and you are always gassy at night. This is common if you consume sodium more than 1000mg a day. With Paleo, the use of sodium and salt is discouraged because of its side effects that cause you to bloat, become gassy, and also unable to burn fat if you are trying to lose weight.

Healthy fats like omega 3 are encouraged in the Paleo diet. The nutritional value of omega 3 has always been immense, but with this diet you intake of this fatty acid increases to exponential levels. Consuming omega 3 regularly benefits your hearth, helps you burn fat quicker, helps you control autoimmune diseases like diabetes, and promotes positive brain development and a much healthier immune system.

Eating un-processed food is the ultimate benefit. This is something that cannot be overlooked about being on a Paleo diet. This diet encourages you to eat natural, organic food, and tells you to avoid harmful processed foods that are full of negative additives, toxins, antibiotics, and growth hormones that are bad for your health anyway. Above all it has a good balance of macronutrient
(protein, carbohydrates, and fats) and their appropriate ratios, which should not only nourish and give you exceptional overall health, but also give you mental clarity and a generally better mood.

You will be in optimum health because you will be consuming many nutrients and Vitamins that contribute to giving you good energy for the day, strengthen your immune system and the good fats in a Paleo diet will help with good health of arteries, maintain good skin and healthy brain function.

When you are on a Paleo diet the fats, and oils you use will not be harmful to your body because the oils used on a Paleo diet tend to be largely stable and don't go rancid like other commercial vegetable and seed oils that go rancid quickly, which brings about a toxicity to the oil that can be damaging to your body and promote negative heart health.

Eating habits really affect your sleep. People on Paleo diet, have a better overall health, this means better gut health, less bloating, less gassiness, water retention and better sleeping patterns. You will sleep better when you aren't troubled by an upset stomach, or the feeling of being bloated.

While, it may be a bit easier to give up savory foods and snacks, it can be much harder and more painful to let go off everyday desserts like muffins, cakes, cookies, and ice cream. There's a whole culture of comfort built around these desserts. Gossiping friends, lovers on a romantic dinner, or a family night of movies and ice cream, how can you make the transition to a better lifestyle easier without sugar, butter, and flour?

Let's take a peek into the world of guilt free Paleo desserts that are healthy but very tasty and scrumptious at the same time. Once you get the idea that healthy and delicious can work in combination, you will be hooked on the Paleo lifestyle forever.

## The Gluten Free Paleo Way That Is Getting Better Day By Day

There had been a time in the not so distant past, when to say the words 'Gluten- Free' pushed weird looks. Questions regularly surfaced about glue, construction, or maybe couponing craft projects or similar ideas as the concept of 'Gluten- Free' was such a new concept. Who might have guessed a miniscule protein in wheat, barley, and rye could cause such havoc for the gut in a few of the people? And who might have imagined a diet without wheat, or where the protein had been separated somehow? Today, not only is the discourse a hot health subject, but more folk are taking a second look into gluten free recipes and exposing a good advantageous Paleo diet. Continuously, with growing abdominal sensitivities like Celiac illness, and other yeast / sugar digestive issues, this Gluten Free Paleo diet has appeared.

Many of us are still undecided precisely what all this means. With every day new options abound for those looking for techniques to try experimenting with this new Paleo way of life.

We are even beginning to see things from boxed mash to baking products with labels announcing themselves 'Gluten-Free' at the food shop. Betty Crocker even has a gluten free cake mix. In under ten years the modern diet has grown to incorporate assorted digestive system sensitivities. In a case of ten years the modern diet has gone from having this subject utterly obscure and off the wall, to having major corner shop chains carry these 'Gluten-Free' diet express products.

From lactose, to peanuts, customers are familiar with seeing divergences and alternative diets and items on the normal menu. Today, many are made to try alternative diets like the Paleo lifestyle to reduce environmental and modern-life perils and symptoms.

Today, many of us choose to try this 'Glute-Free' Paleo diet out. And when folks are selecting alternative diets like Paleo, recipes are changed, influenced, and creativeness is common. From complete obscurity to celebrity overnight, the Gluten-Free Paleo Lifestyle offers a lot of options and variety to delight the pallet. By taking a stress off wheat, barley, and rye, there are several solutions that commonly increase health. One can decide to eliminate carbs all together, focusing upon plants, or seek choices or altered gluten free, dairy free and grain free foods. Frequently a mix of these options create the most inventive, classy, and unique Paleo recipes.

Sources for Gluten-Free Paleo recipes are skyrocketing by the day, too. The most well-known alternative diet recipe advocates include the gluten free girl and the dinner diva - both are so well knowns now that one can simply use those search phrases and find a range of fascinating options and further info.

Cooking books devoted to this alternative Paleo diet are even a main section in most libraries and book stores now. Lots of the recipes have a tendency to focus upon 1 or 2 styles. Most stress either augmenting veggies and fruits or using alternative wheat substitutes. New grains to the modern pallet that have increased in renown with stress on dumping wheat include various kinds of rice and quinoa. While both are technically gluten free, a few individuals may still experience a hypersensitivity to these extra carb centric foods.

Even still, a good quinoa, cranberry, green apple tart salad can be most succulent coupled with a protein-rich solid like salmon and a desert wine. A diet improved with alternative foods can be quite alluring and pleasurable while enlarging anti- oxidizing compounds, adding variety to your menu, and being less complicated on your gastro abdominal system. The sector of gluten free Paleo recipes is offering new choices to normal wheat.

This new Paleo diet or better yet Paleo way of life offers buyers added health benefits, new tastes, textures, and an entire world of colorful ideas. For the regular consumer facing digestive issues day in and day out, a diet with gluten free Paleo recipes and Paleo dessert recipes is improving by the day.

## Paleo & Fiber

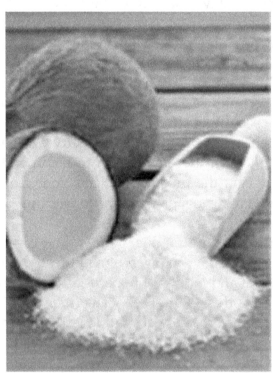

There are some questions that we find come up all the time when we are talking about Paleo. People who are looking make the transit into the paleo lifestyle are always asking us questions related to fiber.

For example, does a Paleo lifestyle provide me with enough fiber because with Paleo there are no grains allowed? People are asking things about whole grains and fiber because they know that these foods do fight cholesterol.

People are confused about the fact that they need a certain amount of fiber into their system in order to stay healthy.

We always get the questions what are the best sources of fiber with the Paleo lifestyle.

People are also not clear about if fiber helps them keep themselves full in order to lose weight when they are on a diet.

All these questions and concerns show how people are unclear and confused about Paleo and fiber and that is the reason why we are dedicating one whole chapter to this topic because it is important to clear up the confusion before we get any further into the main content.

The best way you can start to fix your digestive tract and stomach health is by getting rid of poisonous foods for good: - Cereal grains are bad

- Omega 6 economic seed oils (things like corn, safflower, cottonseed, soybean, and the like) are bad - Processed soy (like soya milk, soy flour and soy protein for example) is bad.

Many people have diverse food sensitivities, with some of the more common perpetrators being dairy and gluten. Removing several these items, and including fermentable foods like kefir, kimchi and sauerkraut may do the job in restoring some healthy tummy bacteria.

You may also help to boost your health by including the right kinds and amounts of fiber. The Institute of Medication commends around thirty-eight grams of fiber for men, and twenty-five grams for girls roughly a day.

Though it isn't wholly important to hit these numbers, a paleo approach to eating will get you extremely close if it does not surpass them. A one thousand calorie portion of fruit and veg will offer you approximately 2 to 7 times the quantity of fiber than whole grains would. And, most this fiber is from soluble sources which are far more favorable in the sense that they feed the healthful bacteria in your stomach.

Soluble fiber ferments in the tummy, and turns into short chain trans-acids that, in turn, help to grow, and feed healthy bacteria. By including more green leafy vegetables, root veg, and tubers like carrots and sweet potato, as well as low sugar fruits like berries, you can add more fiber to your diet, and improve stomach health, but improve mineral and vitamin uptake and assimilation.

Due to phytates and gluten found in foods like beans and numerous wheat-based products, many minerals and vitamins like calcium, iron, and zinc can go unabsorbed. The plants and occasional fruits on a paleo diet supply more than sufficient fiber to your body.

In fact, cups of cooked broccoli would provide you with 7 grams of fiber and only thirty calories, while it would probably take 2 bits of "whole grain" that equal 120 calories to supply the same quantity of fiber.

### Constipation and regular elimination

If staying regular with your guts is an important concern, we suggest first looking at your water consumption. Dehydration or an absence of water is mostly to blame for a poor digestion. It's also possible the grains, dairy, and legumes you were dependent on eating caused leaky tummy. The most effective way to deal with this is by removing food most dangerous to the bowel like commercial seed oils, grains, dairy, and legumes, and by permitting the good bacteria and abdominal flora to reset themselves, and mend the tummy lining. 75 percent of stool is dry weight or dead bacteria, suggesting that fiber isn't required for bulk and elimination.

It can certainly help, but isn't a duty. So long as your body maintains healthy stomach flora, and you steer clear of food that body doesn't endure well, and high fructose foods like honey, soda, agave, breakfast bars and cereals as well as processed junk, you will be able to prevent bowel problems, swelling and gas.

### Fiber supplementation

Many supposed health specialists advocate taking extra fiber products to help with weight management, the lowering of cholesterol, and trots. The issue with this is that your body, or, more particularly, your colonic tract, can become hooked on these products, and need more of them. If you're following a lower carbohydrate diet, and are fighting with the constancy of your stools and cholesterol, first try slowly pushing up your water consumption by roughly 8 oz every day. Then think of adding in more starchy and fermentable foods like sweet potatoes and carrots. Eventually, if those things don't help, or if you have blood sugar issues, and cannot include starchy carbs, give consideration to adding in a soluble fiber supplement like Organic Acacia Fiber, or a prebiotic like Klaire Laboratories Biotagen. In every case, begin reinforcement with a low dose, and steadily increase weekly or bi-weekly.

## Fiber and cholesterol

Fiber and cholesterol This could be the number one thing that frustrates me more than the rest in the world of nourishment.

We just wish to touch on a pair things here. Cholesterol isn't bad. Your body real wants it so as to operate capably. Cholesterol is employed to make cell surfaces, which are used to help each single cell in your body move, and engage with the other cells. The cholesterol you eat has just about nothing to do with the cholesterol in your blood. You eat cholesterol, and create your very own cholesterol each day. Approximately 25 percent of your daily cholesterol is from the food that you eat, and the other 75 percent is basically manufactured by your body. The majority of the cholesterol you eat and produce each day lives in your cell surfaces. It's actually serving a purpose.

Cholesterol in your blood does not imply cholesterol in your arteries. When you get your cholesterol checked, what's measured is the quantity of cholesterol in the blood. The reality is that there is not any way of knowing if that cholesterol is going to finish up in your arteries or not.

Almost all of the cholesterol you eat is pooped out. There's no other way to put it truly. Most cholesterol you eat isn't soaked up - it leaves the body in your stool. Real reasons behind coronary disease are deep set in swelling. This is due generally to the overconsumption of Omega-6 fats from grains, plant oils, and grain-fed animals. One way you may help to combat this is by getting rid of these foods from your diet, and including fitter Omega 3 fats from wild-caught salmon, bolstering with fish oil, and eating more grass-fed meat and lamb.

Rather than counting up fiber grams, mixing up high fibre supplement shakes, taking in nonsensical amounts of grains or legumes, or hunting for fake foods with added fiber, instead get back to eating real food. Stress green leafy plants, lower sugar fruits like berries, and fermentable starchy carbohydrates like sweet potatoes and carrots, increase that water consumption, get routine exercise, and, for Pete's sake, get your rest, and practice correct stress-relieving systems like meditation. Not merely will that keep you regular - it will keep you healthy, content, and fit too.

# Sneak Peak Into The World Of Paleo Desserts

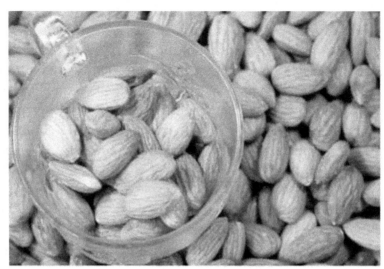

Paleo desserts can be a wondrous world of treats and tastes, if you use the right Paleo ingredients and have yummy recipes on hand to try them. It can be hard to know where to get started when you don't have an idea about Paleo ingredients. After all, what can a cupcake be without milk and sugar? What can a chocolate pudding be without actual chocolate in it? And how can a cheese cake be creamy without a giant helping of cream cheese?

Seems depressing when you think all the flavors you may be missing out on because you're removing all wheat, sugars, and dairy products from your diet. Fear not! There are Paleo substitutes for all those ingredients and more. This chapter will shine a light on all those ingredients, and give you an idea of how to use them compared to conventional ingredients used for desserts.

**Grain free flours:** The key to most desserts is good quality flour. The flour can make or break a cupcake. So, what does Paleo have to offer the texture aficionados of desserts?

**Almond flour:** This is made from finely ground almonds, and gives grainier texture to desserts, but it can be substituted with other flours in a 1:1 ratio. It however, doesn't contain gluten, so while that is good for your health, you may find that it does not provide a dessert with the same elasticity and hold that gluten does with the conventional flours. Not to worry though, you can use this flour for cookies and bakes that need a grainier texture, or substitute slightly with some other Paleo flour for desired texture.

Tips:
Keep in mind also that the finer the almond flour is the better a baked
dessert will turn out.
Keep in mind that nut flour can easily brown, so, keep the heat lower than usual and bake your dessert for longer to compensate for a lower temperature.
Keep the almond flour refriverated, or even frozen and it will last longer.

**Coconut flour:** This is another prized Paleo flour that is approved for dessert making and give batters and desserts a good texture. You can expect a lighter and airier cupcake with this flour. However, coconut flour cannot be substitutes at a 1:1 ratio with other flours because of the rate at which it absorbs liquid. You can substitute about ¼ cups of coconut flour with 1 cup of any other nut based, or grain based flour. With about ½ a cup coconut use 5 eggs and ½ a cup of coconut milk to compensate for the absorbent nature of coconut flour.

Tips:

Try adding mashed fruit for moisture in the baking.

Store your coconut flour at room temperature.

Sift your flour before using it, as it tends to be clumpy.

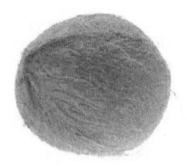

Fats and oil

Choosing a Paleo fat that will both compliment a dessert and not contribute to bad cholesterol isn't hard when it comes to Paleo. Many healthy examples are available that both do justice to a scrumptious dessert recipe and also provide good health benefits.

Use coconut oil and butter in desserts, this is a stable oil at high temperatures and works well in recipes which call for a vegetable oil, or shortening. Earlier concerns of the amount of saturated fats in coconut oil have been outweighed by the benefits of this oil. This oil increases metabolic rate and also contributes positively to the immune system.

Use almond butter, or any other nut butter in your desserts, they add decadence and are creamy and make your baking smell amazing.

Use grass fed butter or ghee in your desserts. Additive and antibiotic free butter and ghee are high in good saturated fats.

Dairy:

Use coconut milk, or almond milk. Both work well in most of the dessert recipes and provide great flavor. Coconut milk gives great coconut cream frosting that tastes amazing when whipped.

### Sweeteners:

There are many Paleo approved sweeteners like medjool dates, grade B maple syrup, and honey that have made the list and can be substituted for sugar in dessert recipes. Raw honey is the best of the list and considered closely approved by the Paleo diet as an organic ingredient that is good for human body and does not exponentially increase blood sugar levels in your body. Dates are great for incorporating sweetness in both baked goods and pudding and ice creams. They provide an amazing amount of sweetness, and are still good for your health.

### Chocolate:

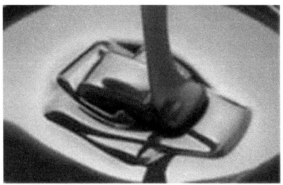

Chocolate cake without cocoa? Chocolate pudding without chocolate? No way! Don't worry, the Paleo diet allows for unsweetened cocoa powder, or raw version of it called cacao powder.
Use dark chocolate with 70% cocoa content, or 85% cocoa content, or use unsweetened dark chocolate.

Paleo Marzipan & Berry Muffins With Coconut Whipped Cream

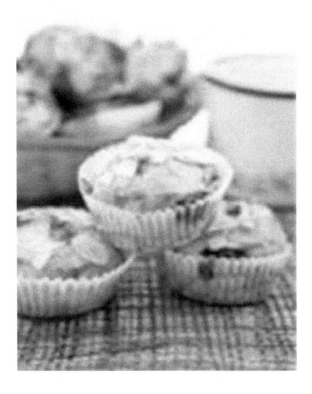

Let's get started so that you get into the mood as well and we hope that our scrumptious Paleo marzipan & blueberry muffins are getting you excited and moving, too.

### Ingredients:

¼ cup of organic coconut flour (buy in health store) ¼ baking power
¼ teaspoon of salt
a dash of organic cinnamon spice
3 fresh farm eggs
2 tablespoon of melted butter (organic if possible) 1 teaspoon of organic vanilla extract
3 tablespoon of organic marzipan
1/2 cup of fresh or frozen blueberries (all organic if possible) Directions:
Heat your cooker to 350 F
Grease your muffin tins with coconut oil and line them with paper If you like to push the easy baking button to save lots of time and money, just use these reusable muffin molds from the Scrumptious & Oozing Baking Kit that you can find here: http://answerszone.info/ILike/scrumptiousoozing
In a huge bowl, mix all of the dry ingredients together: salt, baking powder, coconut flour and cinnamon
In another bowl mix the fresh farm eggs, melted butter, organic vanilla and organic marzipan. Mix them uniformly.
Now mix the ingredients of both the bowls and form a smooth batter Stir all of the blueberries in the batter
Grease the interior of the muffin baking dish and cook for about twenty minutes Your delightful Paleo marzipan blueberry muffins are prepared Ingredients Coconut Whipped Cream 1 can of fat coconut milk (organic if possible) 1 tbsp. of vanilla extract (organic if possible)

### Directions:

Go ahead and mix the ingredients into a fluffy light coconut whipped cream (add some raw honey if you like it sweet) and serve with the paleo marzipan blueberry treats together with a nice mug of freshly brewed coffee, tea, or hot chocolate that fits your brand and flavor

## Flourless Paleo Chocolate Muffins With Coconut Whipped Cream

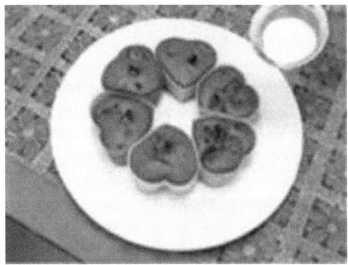

Lets experiment with some exotic ingredients like coconut oil, coconut milk and shredded coconut. This moist, tasty & flourless Paleo choc muffins with coconut whipped cream will motivate your loved ones keep asking you for more of this heavenly delight.

### Ingredients:

1 cup of organic almond flour
¼ teaspoon of baking soda
3 tablespoon of raw organic cacao powder ¼ cup of organic shredded coconut 2 tablespoons of softened organic butter
2 tablespoon of organic coconut oil
11/2 cup of full fat organic coconut milk 1 teaspoon of organic vanilla extract 2 tablespoons of organic raw honey
1 fresh farm egg
Ingredients for the coconut whipped cream frosting: 1 can organic fat coconut milk
1 tablespoon of organic vanilla extract

### Directions:

Mix all your dry ingredients together: organic coconut and raw organic cacao powder In another mixing bowl add all wet ingredients together Now add this to your almond flour mix Fill your paper lined muffin cups with the batter and bake for 350 F for approximately 20 minutes If you like to push the easy baking button to save lots of time and money, just use these reusable muffin molds from the Scrumptious & Oozing Baking Kit that you can find here: http://answerszone.info/ILike/scrumptiousoozing
Cool the muffins on a rack
Top them with your coconut cream frosting and decorate with some toasted shredded coconut and serve Directions Frosting:

Place a can of organic full fat coconut milk in your refrigerator with an open lid This process helps your coconut milk to thicken up and to separate from the coconut water Take the solid coconut material and put it in a mixing bowl Add some organic vanilla extract

Mix everything thoroughly until everything is light and fluffy Take a knife ore a spatula and spread this delicious cream over your muffins Serve as fresh as possible!

### Paleo Black Sesame Coconut Flour Muffins

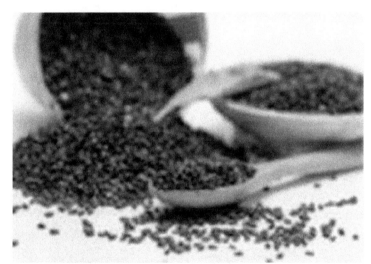

The sound of black sesame coconut might recall some exotic adventures which is exactly what we are looking for as we are experimenting with this paleo muffin recipe: The Black Sesame Coconut Flour Muffins. What is great about it is that it only uses 6 ingredients and these muffins are very high in protein and fiber. It is quick to make, healthy and very scrumptious in taste and thus qualifies to be part of this collection. Let's get started.

### Ingredients:

3 tablespoons of organic black sesame powder 1/4 cup of organic coconut flour 1/4 cup of organic coconut sugar
2 fresh farm eggs
1/4 teaspoon of baking soda 1/2 cup of organic almond milk

### Directions:

Preheat your oven to 180°C (350°F) Grease and line your favorite muffin molds and tin them with paper cases If you like to push the easy baking button to save lots of time and money, just use these reusable muffin molds from the Scrumptious & Oozing Baking Kit that you can find here:

http://answerszone.info/ILike/scrumptiousoozing

In a medium sized baking bowl, add your organic coconut flour, your organic black sesame powder, and your organic coconut sugar, and finally the baking soda In another mixing bowl, mix together the fresh farm eggs and organic almond milk Stir this batter into your dry ingredients Lastly, divide your batter and fill your greased muffin tins Bake the muffins for approximately 30 minutes Test with a toothpick and if the tops are firm to the touch you can cool them on a rack Serve them oven fresh with some paleo cream or natural like this

## Macadamia, White Chocolate & Raspberry Muffins

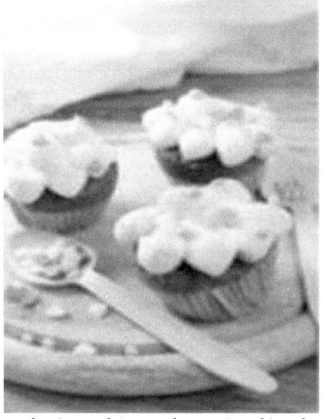

We love these Paleo macadamia raspberry and organic white chocolate muffins so much because the combination of the white chocolate with the raspberries and the nutty touch of the macadamia is almost perfection. So let's get going with this scrumptious treat. We promise you one result with this one and that is one resounding: "Can I get more?"

### Ingredients:

2 fresh farm eggs
2 cups of organic almond flour
¼ cup of organic raw honey
¼ cup of organic coconut oil
1 tablespoon of organic vanilla extract

1 teaspoon of organic apple cider vinegar ¼ teaspoon of baking soda
¼ teaspoon of sea salt
cup of organic white chocolate chips 1 cup of organic and fresh or organic and frozen raspberries

Directions:

Preheat your oven to 350F
Mix all your dry and the wet ingredients separately Exclude your fresh or frozen raspberries and your organic chocolate chips After the batter is done, make sure to add in the chocolate chips and the raspberries Next, bake your muffins by either using a well-greased paper lined muffin tins Or use your favorite silicone muffin molds because they do not need any greasing and fooling around with paper liners Bake your muffins for around 15 to 20 minutes and check with a toothpick Cool them on a rack and serve oven fresh You might add a decorative raspberry on top of each muffin that you serve.

Banana Nut Paleo Muffins

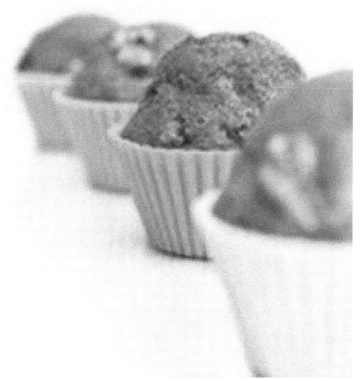

Today finding scrumptious recipes for the Paleo lifestyle has become stylish for health aware people and those with delicate digestive tracts around the globe so here is yet another great Paleo muffin recipes that you might enjoy in harmony with your partner while respecting the rules of Paleo.

## Ingredients:

4 fresh farm eggs
1/2 cup of organic almond butter
2 tablespoons of organic coconut oil
1 teaspoon of organic vanilla extract
1/2 cup of organic coconut flour 1/2 teaspoon of nutmeg spice
2 teaspoons of cinnamon spice 1 teaspoon of baking powder 1 teaspoon of baking soda
1/4 teaspoon of salt
4 small and ripe organic bananas (mash the bananas with a fork and the more
ripe the bananas the better)

## Directions:

Preheat your oven to 350 degrees F
Grease and line your favorite muffin tin with cups or use your favorite reusable muffin molds
Use a large mixing bowl and combine: the mashed bananas, the fresh farm eggs, the organic
almond butter, the organic coconut oil, and lastly the organic vanilla extract Using your favorite
hand blender, blend everything together until well combined Next, add organic coconut flour,
the cinnamon and nutmeg spice, the baking soda, the baking powder and finally the salt Blend
the dry ingredients into the wet mixture of ingredients Divide your batter into your lined muffin
tins and fill two-thirds of the way full Finally, go ahead and bake your muffins for
approximately 20 to 25 minutes Use a toothpick and see if it comes out clean Serve this
deliciousness oven warm. If you have some paleo ice cream you can put a scoop of paleo banana
ice cream or any other favored ice cream made the paleo way on the side.

## The Ultimate Paleo Cocoholic's Muffins

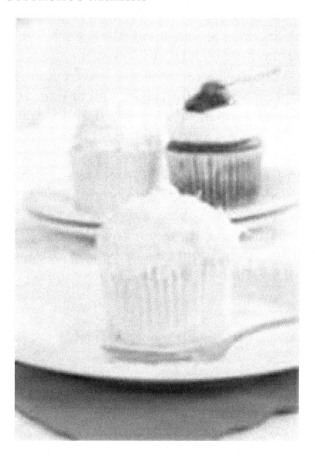

These scrumptious Cocoholic Muffins are very tempting and in our humble opinion this recipe should not miss on any mom's dinner table. It is simple to make, but wicked in taste! Serve these at the end of a nice dinner and your loved one will be happy happy happy!

### Paleo Muffins:

2 tablespoon of organic coconut flour
1/3 cup of organic almond flour
2 tablespoons of arrowroot flour
1/4 teaspoon of baking powder 1/8 teaspoon of sea salt
3/4 cup of organic berries (fresh or frozen)
3 fresh farm eggs
3 ½ tablespoons of organic coconut sugar crystals 2 tablespoons of coconut oil (organic if possible) 1 tablespoon of vanilla extract (organic if possible)

### Directions:

Go ahead and preheat your oven to 350 degrees F

Next, take a mixing bowl and combine your dry ingredients: coconut flour, almond flour, arrowroot flour and finally your baking powder Mix until combined

Combine your farm eggs, the organic coconut sugar, the sea salt, the organic coconut oil and the organic vanilla extract in your favorite blender (We are using the Nutribullet for this recipe)

Add your wet ingredients to your dry ingredients and fold in your fresh or frozen berries

Grease your traditional muffin molds with the coconut oil or line each one with a paper liner If you like to push the easy baking button to save lots of time and money, just use these reusable muffin molds from the Scrumptious & Oozing Baking Kit that you can find here: http://answerszone.info/ILike/scrumptiousoozing

Fill each muffin mold almost all the way to the top Take another bowl and combine: your tablespoon of organic shredded and unsweetened coconut, one tablespoon of organic coconut sugar crystals, one teaspoon of cinnamon spice and go ahead and sprinkle this blend on top of the muffins and before you put them into the oven. You'll soon see and smell the delicious crust. You can take out your muffins after 15 minutes of baking Use a toothpick to test if they are baked Serve oven fresh and if you like you can put a little whipped coconut cream on the side.

Red Berries & White Chocolate Paleo Muffins

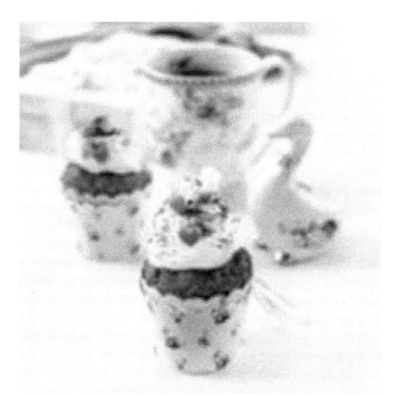

Like raspberries, strawberries work perfectly in combination with white chocolate and both strawberries and raspberries round up the meal. In this case we picked both raspberries and strawberries in combination with some other red fruits that you can find already packed and frozen. You can find organic frozen berry mixes and this is what we use here. This is an old traditional family recipe from Germany that we transformed into the Paleo way of making desserts. We kept the measures original and authentic.

Ingredients:

150 gram of organic almond meal 160 gram of organic coconut flour 150 gram of organic almond meal 200 gram of organic almond milk 2 fresh farm eggs
25 gram of organic agave syrup
80 gram of organic macadamia oil
a dash of baking powder
100 gram of organic fresh or frozen red mixed berries 200 gram of white chocolate (sugar free and organic)

### Directions:

Preheat your oven to around 180 degrees
Place all your above ingredients with the exception of the red mixed berries and the organic white chocolate into a large mixing bowl Mix all ingredients together for approximately 1 to 2 minutes and on speed level 5 of your blender Next, add your red mixed berries and your organic unsweetened white chocolate into the batter and go ahead and whisk for another minute on a lower speed Grease your traditional muffin molds with some coconut oil or line each one with a paper liner Divide your batter into the molds and bake your muffins for approximately 25 to 30 minutes at 350 degrees F
Remove them from the oven and cool them on a rack Serve oven fresh with some cream on the side and decorate with the remaining red fruits.


### Paleo Lemon Chia Seed Muffins


Paleo Lemon Chia Seed Muffins are not only very scrumptious but very low carb, dairy, grain and nut free. This is a totally gluten-free and refined sugar-free Paleo dessert that not only tastes good but it is a guilt free pleasure for someone who is on a diet This dessert can be enjoyed in a guilt free way and no sacrifices have to be made.


### Ingredients:

1 tablespoon of organic chia seeds
⅓ cup of organic coconut flour
¼ cup of organic tapioca flour
2 tablespoons of organic coconut oil (make sure it is melted) ¼ teaspoon of salt
⅛ teaspoon of baking soda
½ cup of organic coconut milk 3 fresh farm eggs
3 tablespoons of organic maple syrup 1 tablespoon of organic lemon juice 1 teaspoon of organic vanilla extract
2 teaspoons of organic lemon zest


### Directions:


Mix together your organic coconut flour, your organic tapioca flour, your baking soda, your organic chia seeds and the salt Take another mixing bowl and mix together the organic coconut oil, the organic coconut milk, the farm eggs, your organic maple syrup, the lemon zest and the juice and finally the organic vanilla extract Mix your wet and dry ingredients together until they combine well into a nice batter Grease your traditional muffin molds with some coconut oil or line each one with a paper liner or use your favorite silicone baking molds Next divide your batter into the cups Bake at for 30 to 35 minutes at 350 degrees F and until the muffin tops are golden brown Let the muffins cool off on a wire rack Serve with some organic lemon preserve or jam on the side These also make great breakfast muffins with a cup of zesty lemon tea or a nice cup of Earl Grey.

### Paleo Choc Hazelnut Muffins

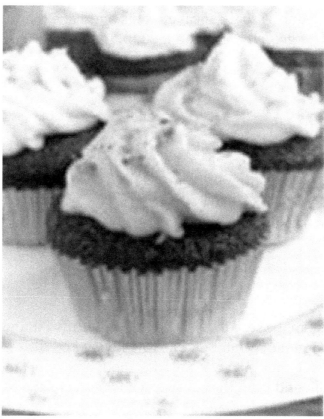

The Paleo Choc Hazel Muffins consist of a creamy dark chocolate topping which perfectly blends with the scrumptious & oven warm nut flavor of the hazelnuts. Be careful because these delicious muffins will not last very long if you do not keep an eye on them.

Ingredients:

1 package of the brand called Paleo Baking Company Hazelnut Cake & Muffin Mix or a similar brand
6 fresh farm eggs
1 cup of liquid organic coconut oil (make sure it is melted)
1 cup of raw organic honey
1/2 cup of warm water
3 oz. 72% dark organic chocolate (chopped into chunks)

### Directions:

The most important thing here is that you go ahead and read the instructions on your package of the Paleo Muffin Mix and follow through according to the instructions Combine all your wet ingredients before you are adding the dry mix Next and once everything is combined go ahead and add your chopped dark

organic chocolate Grease your traditional muffin molds with some coconut oil or line each one with a paper liner If you like to push the easy baking button to save lots of time and money, just use these reusable muffin molds from the Scrumptious & Oozing Baking Kit that you can find here: http://answerszone.info/ILike/scrumptiousoozing

Divide your batter into the individual cupcake molds and bake the muffins 20 to 25 minutes at 350 degrees They should be golden brown on the top and firm to the touch Remove them from the oven

Cool them off on a wire rack

### Paleo Chocolate Topping Ingredients:

1 to 2 tablespoons of organic coconut milk 2 cups solid organic coconut oil
1 cup of raw organic honey
1       cup of raw organic cocoa powder

### Directions:

Before you do the frosting, make sure to chill your hazel muffins in the fridge for approximately 30 minutes Combine the organic coconut oil, the raw honey and the organic cocoa powder and 1 tablespoon of your coconut milk in your favorite food processor and mix until smooth Add more organic coconut milk and until the consistency is perfect Take a knife or spatula and frost the chilled muffins Serve them immediately

Top the muffins with chopped dark organic chocolate and chopped hazelnuts We love to serve either a fresh brew of hazelnut tea or coffee with this scrumptious delight!

### Paleo Blueberry Delights

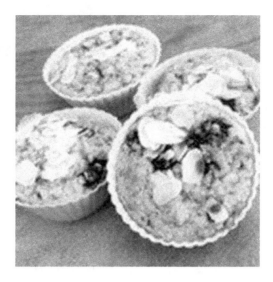

This fruity Blueberry delight treat is something for blueberry lovers. If you love your cake moist, you'll like this moist tartness of this blueberry muffin dessert.

For this recipe, we love to use organic frozen blueberries in the muffins. If you like you can substitute other red berries or other chopped stone fruits instead of the blueberries.

You can also substitute more fruits for the sugar. Some bakers are trying to avoid adding any additional sweeteners to their baked goods which is fine and you can use raw honey or fruits instead of sugar.

These raspberry treats are low on fructose and gluten free.

Ingredients:

1/2 cup of organic coconut flour 1/3 cup of organic coconut sugar 1 cup of organic almond flour
2 teaspoons of baking powder
150 gram of frozen or fresh blueberries
2 large farm eggs
1 1/3 cup of organic almond milk

Directions:

Preheat your oven to 180°C (350°F)

Grease and line your favorite muffin molds and tin them with paper cases if you like or use your favorite reusable silicone muffin molds Mix all your dry ingredients in a baking bowl Take a second mixing bowl and whisk together your farm eggs and the organic almond milk Stir the wet batter into your dry ingredients Fold in your blueberries or other red fruits You do not need to defrost your berries if you are using frozen fruits Lastly, evenly divide and distribute the batter into your muffin molds Bake the muffins for approximately 30 minutes and until they are golden in color and firm in touch Remove them from the oven and cool them on a wire rack Make sure to serve this deliciousness oven warm with a little whipped coconut cream and the rest of the berries on the side You can also serve some almond cream on the top.

Some additional baking tips:
Substitute, for example 1 small ripe organic banana or 1/4 cup of organic apple or organic pear puree if you'd like to add some more sweetness to these baked goods then add these fruits to your wet ingredients
Blend your batter until everything is combined well mixed Please go ahead and substitute the organic almond milk with another organic coconut milk or another type of milk and to your preferences

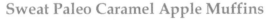

Sweat Paleo Caramel Apple Muffins

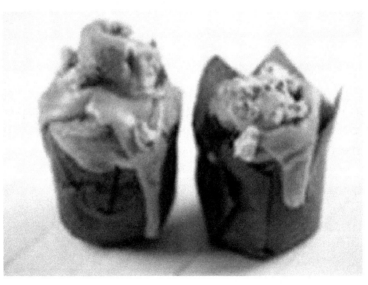

These Paleo Caramel dessert muffins are gluten free and free from starch.

Ingredients for the Coconut Caramel Sauce:

1 can of full fat, organic & unsweetened coconut milk 1/4 cup of pure and organic maple syrup or organic raw honey if you prefer 1/4 cup of organic coconut sugar
1 teaspoon of pure and organic vanilla extract 1/2 teaspoon of coarse sea salt
1 tablespoon of organic unsalted butter

### Directions:

Mix your organic coconut milk, the organic maple syrup or the raw honey, and your organic coconut palm sugar in a medium saucepan and over medium high heat Bring the mix to a boil and boil it until thickened and amber in color It should be reduced to 1 to 1 1/4 cups
Once you got this desired consistency mix in the organic vanilla, the salt and the unsalted organic butter Cool this mix completely
You can use this mix or store it refrigerated for around 3 weeks Caramel Apple

### Sauce Directions:

Combine 1/4 cup of this caramel sauce and one organic apple that is very finely cut Use a medium sauce pan for this
Simmer over a medium heat until your apple is tender Cool the mix and puree this mix in order to create your caramel apple sauce Coconut Caramel Apple Muffins.

### Ingredients:

16 gram of organic coconut flour
96 gram of organic almond flour
1/8 teaspoon of salt
1/2 teaspoon of garam masala, alternatively you can also use organic cinnamon or organic pumpkin pie spice, too 1 teaspoon of baking powder (we also suggest Bakewell starch that is starch free baking powder) 1/4 cup of organic and melted coconut oil
3 tablespoons of organic and raw honey 1 teaspoon of organic vanilla extract
3 fresh farm eggs
1/2 cup of finely sliced organic apples
1/2 cup of caramel apple sauce from above

### Directions:

Preheat your oven to 375 degrees and grease your muffin molds and line them with papers If you like to push the easy baking button to save lots of time and money, just use these reusable muffin molds from the Scrumptious & Oozing Baking Kit that you can find here: http://answerszone.info/ILike/scrumptiousoozing

Put together all your dry ingredients in medium mixing bowl Next, combine your wet ingredients in a second baking bowl Add your wet ingredients into your dry ingredients and whisk until combined Distribute the mixture into your muffin molds Bake the muffins approximately 15-20 minutes

Cool them on a wire rack

Serve these muffin treats oven fresh and warm with a topping of our lovely caramel sauce and a nice slice of apple which gives this trat an extra scrumptious flavor We love to brew a strong blend of organic apple cinnamon tea and serve the muffins together with this hot beverage

Mini Blueberry Bites

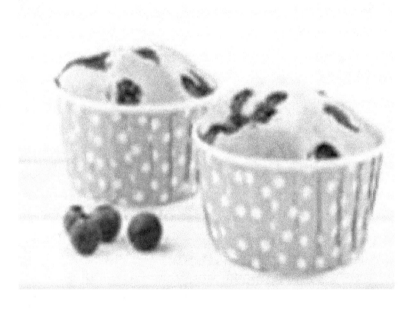

This recipe is perfect for someone who is on a Paleo diet with cravings for some sweet delights. This recipe is totally safe and paleo diet approved so that you can enjoy sweets the guilt free way!

Ingredients:

3 tablespoons of organic raw honey

3 fresh farm eggs

2 tablespoons of melted organic coconut oil 2 tablespoons of organic coconut or organic almond milk and whatever milk you prefer 1/4 teaspoon of salt

1/4 teaspoon of organic vanilla extract 1/4 teaspoon of organic baking powder 1/4 cup of organic coconut flour

1 cup of organic fresh or frozen blueberries

## Directions:

Preheat your oven to approximately 400 degrees Add your fresh farm eggs, your organic coconut oil, your raw honey, your organic milk, your salt and finally your organic vanilla extract and mix until smooth Combine your baking powder and your organic coconut flour Do this before you add the flour into the wet mixture Combine the ingredients together until they combine into a nice batter and before folding in your blueberries Finally, fold in the blueberries in a delicate way Distribute your batter into your prepared muffin molds Bake the muffins for approximately 10 minutes Check with a toothpick and if it comes out clean your muffins are ready Let them cool on a wire rack

Serve them oven fresh and with a fluffy whipped cream on the side We love to serve a hot and strong blend of organic blueberry tea with cream (coconut or almond).

### Paleo Pineapple, Ginger & Passionfruit Cupcakes

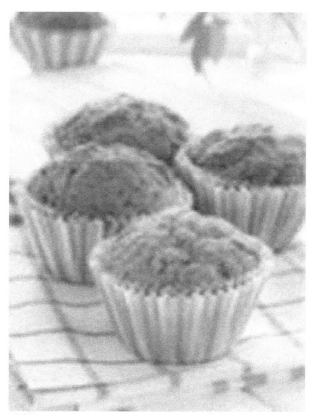

Now let us see how to make some zesty spiced up ginger, pineapple and passion fruit paleo cupcakes.

### Ingredients:

2 passion fruits (make sure to cut them in half) 225 g of organic pineapple pieces (buy it fresh and cut it up or find an organic brand with pineapple chunks)
2 tablespoon of organic coconut flour

1/3 cup of organic almond flour
1 teaspoon of raw honey
3/4 cups of organic coconut milk
1 fresh farm egg
1/2 cup of organic almond oil 3/4 organic marzipan
1 teaspoon of ground ginger spice
2 tablespoon of desiccated coconut (organic if possible)
2 tablespoons of coconut milk

Directions:

Preheat your oven to 350 degrees F
Mix the organic flour, honey, ginger, marzipan and organic coconut together in a mixing bowl
Make a depth in the center.
Add your organic coconut milk, your organic almond oil, half of the passion fruit, the pineapple chunks plus some extra organic coconut milk Mix all the ingredients until smooth Lime some small 2 tablespoon capacity flat based patty pans with paper liners Evenly distribute the batter Bake the cupcakes for approximately 15 - 20 minutes Let them cool off on a wire rack
Serve them oven fresh with a little whipped coconut cream on top

Paleo Chocolate Pot De Crème

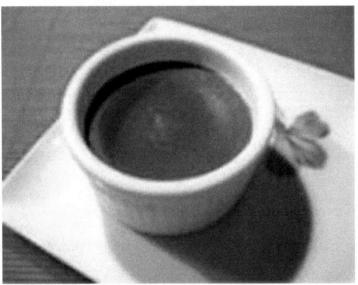

Even though every day is a special day in our home, we like to share this special dessert recipe with bakers who do appreciate a truly special dessert.
It is not only special, but truly decadent because it is full of rich chocolate.
It is a must have for chocolate lovers who appreciate a perfect chocolate perfection the Paleo way.

### Ingredients:

1 cup of organic coconut milk
6 oz of 70% dark chocolate (chop it into bite chunks) 2 fresh farm eggs
1 teaspoon of organic vanilla extract a couple of fresh and organic raspberries for the decoration.

### Directions:

Take a baking bowl and add your dark chopped chocolate, the fresh eggs, and your organic vanilla extract Blend everything in a high-power blender until the texture is very smooth Take a saucepan and heat up the organic coconut milk until to a point where it is almost boiling Make sure that it does not bubble yet

Pour the organic coconut milk into your high-speed blender Blend the mixture until everything is smooth Place 4 organic raspberries in the bottom of 4 8 oz reusable muffin molds or pots or other adequate dishes like soufflé dishes Pour the rich chocolate cream mixture into your molds or dishes and over the fresh raspberries Cover each dish so that it is closed.

Go ahead and chill the Chocolate Pot de Cremes in your fridge and until they are cold Before serving make sure to decorate them with some shaved organic dark chocolate, some fresh raspberries and offer some extra whipped coconut cream in a separate bowl so that your guests can help themselves. You can offer some chilled or hot drinks that match this rich chocolaty flavor. We love to indulge ourselves with some chilled Amaretto and for those who do not drink liquor we like to offer some chilled alcohol free beverages, or a nice blend of freshly brewed almond tea with a splash of coconut cream. A nice cup of hot cocoa made from organic and raw cocoa powder is always welcome by the kids.

## Lemon Coconut Macadamia Muffins

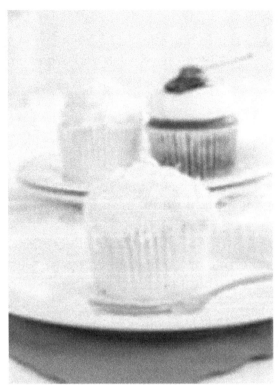

If you are looking for something with flavor this is your recipe because the rich taste of the blueberries in combination with the lemon and nuts is like a burst of sweet deliciousness. The recipe is based on the natural sweetness that is contained in the organic coconut cream and in the blueberry fruits. The recipe is totally free from dairy, grain, sugar and it is gluten free, too.

Ingredients:

1 cup of organic coconut cream (it is the coconut concentrate or coconut butter) 1/4 cup of organic macadamia nut oil (alternatively you can also use organic coconut oil) 6 pastured eggs (organic if possible)
3/4 teaspoons of baking soda 1/2 teaspoon of sea salt
the juice of 1/2 organic squeezed lemon the zest of one organic lemon
3/4 cups of organic fresh or frozen blueberries 1/2 cup of organic macadamia nuts (chopped)

Directions:

Preheat your oven to 180°C (350°F)
Grease and line your favorite muffin molds and tin them with paper cases If you like to push the easy baking button to save lots of time and money, just use these reusable muffin molds from the Scrumptious & Oozing Baking Kit that you can find here: http://answerszone.info/ILike/scrumptiousoozing

Combine your eggs, your organic coconut cream concentrate, your organic macadamia nut oil, your baking soda, and your sea salt until the mixture is very smooth Everything should be well combined.

Use your favorite food processor, mixer or blender for this Add the organic lemon juice and the organic lemon zest to the batter Next go ahead and pour your batter into a baking bowl and fold in the organic fresh or frozen blueberries and the organic chopped macadamia nuts in a very delicate way Distribute your batter into your prepared muffin molds and fill each cup about 3/4 full Bake your muffins for 35-45 minutes

A golden-brown top shows you that they are ready Cool them on a wire rack

We prefer to serve them oven warm because their flavor comes out so deliciously.

You can add some more scrumptiousness by adding some almond butter or cream, or some fluffy whipped coconut cream or some organic ghee if you like the Eastern kitchen and philosophy like we do!

Strawberry Ricotta Paleo Cupcakes

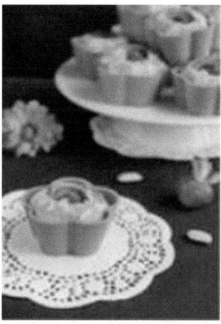

Paleo cupcake recipes are easy to make and the following desssert is good for you, too!

Strawberries and ricotta cheese can be incorporated to make this great cupcake that is rich in antioxidants, high in protein, and a bit of coconut oil keeps everything perfectly balanced and moist.

This recipe is a perfect way of satisfying that four o'clock craving for something sweet. It is not sugary, but there is an underlying sweetness which is fairly addictive.

In this recipe, almond flour is used. Almond flour is tasty and high in nutrients. Apart from a huge dose of polyunsaturated fatty acids and Omega 6, which are very good for your body, it is low in carbohydrates and rich in protein.

Coconut flour is high in fiber and proteins. It is a perfect substitute for flour, and supplies the body with Lauric acid. Lauric acid helps boost the immune system, and improves the quality of your skin.

Strawberries are heavy in antioxidants and vitamins, and raw honey provides the sweetness. Honey is a natural sweetener, but you can substitute it with agave nectar or coconut nectar, as per your liking. Honey is great for your digestion and skin.

Eggs add the extra protein, and a further addition of ricotta cheese makes this a high-protein, low-carb treat that will keep you feeling full and satisfied.

Although dairy is not generally added in Paleo diet, it is a good way of adding some probiotics to your meals which can be considered good for your tummy.

### Ingredients:

150 gm. almond flour 75 gm. coconut flour
150 ml. raw honey or coconut nectar 2 free range organic eggs 1 teaspoon baking powder
1 pinch salt
75 ml. coconut oil, melted 6 strawberries, pureed
Ingredients for the Icing:
100 gm. Ricotta Cheese
50 ml. raw honey or coconut nectar
2 drops vanilla extract

### Directions:

Sift together the almond flour, coconut flour, salt and baking powder Mix together the raw honey with coconut oil, strawberry puree and eggs together Whisk the mixture well to incorporate the honey, and then combine with the dry ingredients Pour in 12 individual cupcake molds, lined with cupcake liners, till the liner is 3/4th full Put the pan in a preheated 180 degree centigrade oven Bake for 15-18 minutes, depending on your oven's temperature, till the cupcakes are done (a toothpick should come out holding moist crumbs when inserted in the center of a cupcake).

Let cool for an hour before icing

For the icing, put the cheese, honey and vanilla in a food processor and process till smooth

Spread on top of each cupcake

Paleo Pink Champagne Cupcakes

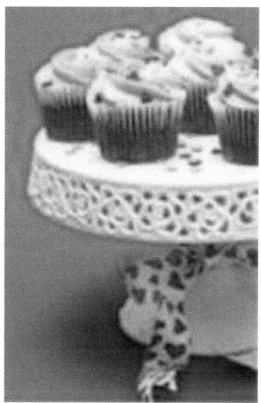

This one is a very special Paleo dessert treat and it is perfect for that special day that you want to celebrate with your loved ones.

Ingredients:

1 teaspoon of organic apple cider vinegar
1 tablespoon of organic soymilk
1-1/4 cups of organic gluten free flour (you can alternatively use the Better Batter Gluten Free Flour brand) 2-1/2 tablespoons of organic coconut four 3/4 teaspoon of baking soda
3/4 teaspoon of baking powder 1/4 teaspoon of salt
1/3 cup coconut oil
raw and organic honey to your taste 1 teaspoon of organic and pure vanilla extract 1 cup of your favorite pink champagne

Directions:

Mix the soymilk and the organic vinegar and set the mixture on the side Whisk the above mix plus the organic coconut oil, the raw honey, the organic and pure vanilla extract.
Add your favorite champagne in a slow way Sift in your organic and gluten free flour, your coconut flour, your baking soda and baking powder and your salt Mix until no big lumps remain in the batter Fill your cups and bake the cupcakes approximately 18 to 20 minutes and at 325 degrees F

Check with a toothpick and if it comes out clean your cupcakes are ready Cool the cupcakes on a wire rack

### Chocolate Champagne Frosting Ingredients:

½ cup of non-dairy and organic butter sticks raw and organic honey 1/2 to 1 cup of raw organic cocoa powder ½ cup of pink champagne

### Directions:

Go ahead and cream your organic no dairy butter Beat in the honey and the organic cocoa and alter with the champagne Spread your cupcakes with the frosting and garnish each cupcake with an organic chocolate dipped strawberry and put it on top of each cupcake Enjoy this scrumptious Champagne delight with a glass of pink Champagne to celebrate a happy happy happy day!

### Scrumptious No Bake Paleo Cakes

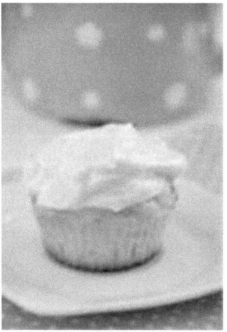

The gluten free Paleo lifestyle truly offers numerous choices and variety to delight any pallet. Some pastry chefs focus upon augmenting fruits as a technique of compensating for the absence of wheat.

Others opt to invent and depend on altered foods that either do not have gluten, or have the key protein removed. With both trying alternative foods and rocketing the amount and spread of fruits, the health is certain to improve.

The basic crux of this alternative Paleo lifestyle is to dump wheat and increase plants.

Ingredients:

Crust:
1 1/2 tablespoon organic raw pure unsweetened cocoa powder 4 medjool organic pitted dates (the dates should be pitted) 1/2 tablespoon of organic coconut oil
3/4 cup of organic unsweetened coconut flakes (alternatively you can also use 1/4 cup of organic coconut flakes and 1/2 cup of organic walnuts) 1/8 teaspoon salt

Filling:
1 small ripe organic banana
1/4 cup of full fat organic coconut milk
1/3 cup of organic coconut butter (organic coconut cream concentrate) 1/4 cup of organic coconut oil
1/8 teaspoon of salt
1 teaspoon of organic vanilla extract
1/2 tablespoon of raw and organic honey (alternatively you can also use pure and organic maple syrup)

Directions:

For the crust:
Preheat your oven to 180°C (350°F)
Grease and line your favorite muffin molds and tin them with paper cases if you like If you like to push the easy baking button to save lots of time and money, just use these reusable muffin molds from the Scrumptious & Oozing Baking Kit that you can find here: http://answerszone.info/ILike/scrumptiousoozing.
Add the crust ingredients to a food processor and blend until you get a batter that is crumbly and coarse in consistency (you can always add more raw and organic cocoa powder to the batter if you like) Distribute the batter into your muffin molds and about 1/2 tablespoon of filling into each muffin cup Press your filling into the bottom of your cups to create a crust If there remains some extra filling, make your crust a little bit thicker.

For the filling:
Heat your organic coconut butter.
Add your remaining ingredients from the list above and process everything in a blender Add the warmed organic coconut butter and the organic coconut milk to the mixer and go ahead and process until everything is very smooth Distribute this batter into your cups and over the crusts Freeze your cups for an hour or for two hours and until everything is very firm Remove the no bake cakes from your muffin cups Store the no bake muffins in your fridge or freezer Serve them chilled like this or allow them to soften a bit for 5 to 15 minutes before serving For the decoration you can drizzle some raw organic chocolate on top of the no bake cakes

### Directions for the organic chocolate drizzle:

Melt approximately 1/4 cup of raw &organic chocolate chips in a saucepan You can also go ahead and melt some raw and organic chopped chocolate in the microwave at 10 to 30 second intervals or you can do this alternatively in a double boiler on your stove Add one tablespoon of organic coconut oil.

You can also go ahead and mix equal parts of raw organic cocoa powder and pure raw honey, a pinch of salt and of organic coconut oil Sprinkle this paleo chocolate drizzle over the tops of your scrumptious no bake cakes after taking them out of your fridge or freezer A nice hot cup of freshly brewed organic and flavored coffee or tea makes this no bake treat a delight that combines a palatable sensation of hot and cold.

Coconut Almond Paleo Smoothie

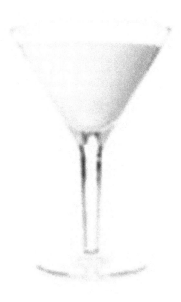

Ingredients:

1/2 cup of organic Almond Milk 1 extra small ripe banana (organic) 1 organic lime (juiced) 1/4 cup of organic & salted macadamia nuts
2 tablespoons of organic cacao nibs
1 tablespoon of organic coconut palm sugar 2 teaspoon of cinnamon spice (organic) some ice cubes and to your liking

Directions:

Add all the above ingredients into your favorite blender Blend until smooth Enjoy!

Creamy Paleo Coconut Macadamia Coffee Smoothie

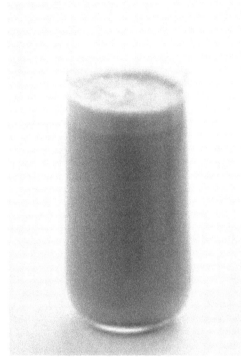

The Paleo diet is one of the healthiest diet options that has many health benefits. One thing that people following a paleo diet often complain about is the fact that they cannot indulge in their favorite desserts and smoothies while following this diet. There is no need to worry anymore. You can simply alter some ingredients of the smoothies like dairy products and sugar. You can consume a vast variety of smoothies that are not only delicious but also Paleo proven. Hence, the next time you throw a party you can serve healthy smoothies as desserts to your friends as yet another healthy dessert option.

Ingredients:

3/4 cup of organic coconut milk 1/2 cup of cold organic coffee 1/4 cup of organic avocado 1/4 cup of organic macadamia nuts 1/4 cup of ice cubes
2 scoops of stevia or raw organic honey to the taste.

Directions:

Add all the ingredients into the blender and blend until a smooth consistency is attained Garnish it with a few macadamia nuts and almond flakes for an added texture This smoothie is also a great idea as a low carb breakfast recipe as it uses coconut milk instead of full fat milk and uses stevia which is a low calorie substitute for sugar. If you do not like the idea of stevia you can instead use raw organic honey Hence this is also a dairy free and gluten free breakfast recipe that you can enjoy together with the person that is closest to your heart!

Creamy Coconut Maca Raw Chocolate Paleo Smoothie

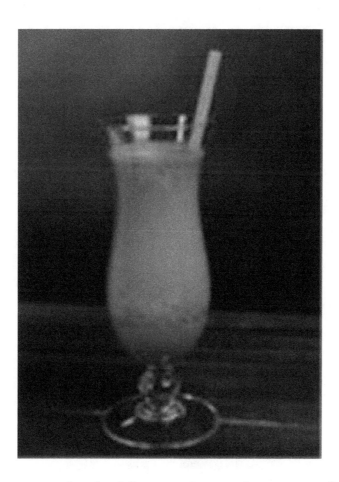

This smoothie recipe has a great depth of flavor as it uses cinnamon and vanilla and poppy seed paste.
This smoothie recipe is a great option for paleo smoothie recipes. Not only is it absolutely incredible to the taste, but also extremely healthy as the ingredients are picked keeping the paleo diet in mind.

Ingredients

1 cup of organic coconut water
1/2 cup of almond milk
1 small frozen and ripe banana
1 tablespoon of raw unsweetened cocoa powder
1 teaspoon of macadamia powder
1/2 teaspoon of organic poppy seed paste 1/2 tea spoon of pure organic vanilla paste 1/2 teaspoon of organic cinnamon spice
1 tablespoon of desiccated coconut

Directions:

Blend all the ingredients until the desired consistency is attained Transfer the smoothie to the serving glass and garnish with macadamia nuts and desiccated coconut on top

Chocolate Cocoa Macadamia Coffee Smoothie

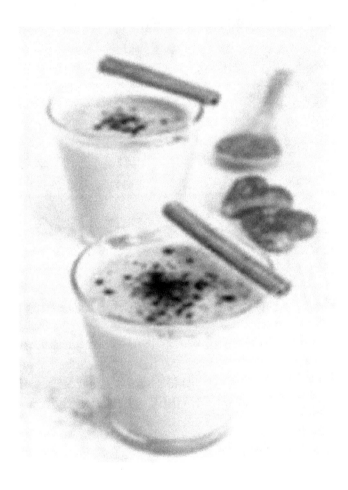

Another smoothie recipe which is a hot favorite for paleo smoothie recipes is the chocolate cocoa macadamia coffee smoothie. The recipe has a very rich texture with a mild flavor. Also considering the recipe uses fat free frozen yogurt instead of ice cream, one can happily enjoy this recipe while keeping the extra calories at bay.

Ingredients:

2 small and ripe organic bananas
1 cup of fat free frozen yogurt (organic if possible) 1/2 cup of organic chilled coffee
1 cup of almond milk
2 tablespoons of unsweetened and organic cocoa powder 1 cup of light whipped coconut cream

Directions:

Add all the smoothie ingredients except the whipped cream to a blender and blend till everything becomes smooth and creamy Transfer the smoothie to a serving glass and top it with the light whipped coconut cream, but if you would like to keep the flavor of the coffee pure you can also enjoy the smoothie without the extra coconut topping!

## Conclusion

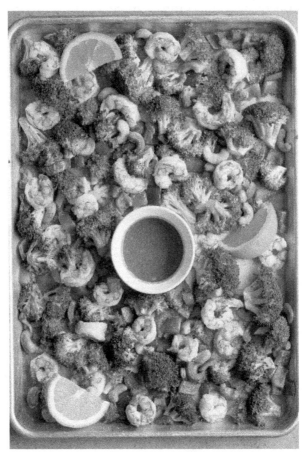

As you can see, dessert recipes are meant to liven the tastes, surprise even the most complex pallet, and even offer increased nourishment, just like the ones you just went through. The choice of the world of Paleo desserts and its ensuing cookbooks is getting bigger and more grand by the day. This awesome Paleo diet and way of life offers health benefits like increased anti oxidizing compounds, new textures and tastes, and a colorful arena of new baking and dessert recipe concepts.

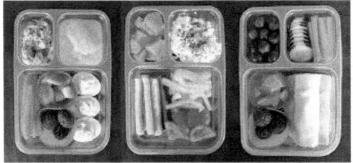

By any standards, the arena of gluten free, grain free and dairy free Paleo recipes is expanding and improving lives every day.

Finding the right kind of dessert that appeases your taste buds should not be a problem with the decadent examples of desserts that can be whipped up with Paleo ingredients. Not only are they fresh, but these recipes are quick and easy to make even for the busiest of the busy people.

This book was meant to give you a peek into the world of Paleo desserts, and these recipes are by no means the complete look at the versatility of Paleo ingredients. Paleo might be somewhat limited approved ingredients, but it is by no means limited in providing taste to your favorite desserts.

Making the change over to a Paleo way of life can be a big change and can take some getting just to, but the health benefits are unrivaled and far greater than not accepting the challenge and putting your health before processed food cravings.

The 'craze' of Paleo as you will discover with your increased knowledge of the Paleo diet is not just a craze, or a fad diet that will eventually melt away into the unknown depths of forgotten failed diet fads. Paleo is here to stay and steadily rising in popularity. What you can do to get a better feel of what you are getting into is gain as much knowledge of the ingredients and Paleo concepts that bring about that wonderful change in your life that everyone else who has been getting positive results from the Paleo lifestyle has been experiencing.

Hopefully by now you do understand the true significance and meaning of the Paleo lifestyle and hopefully you can see what the Paleo lifestyle can do for your own health and happiness.

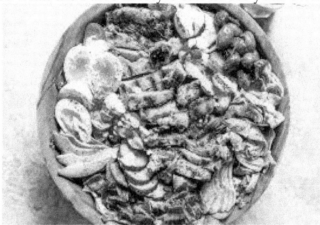

As mentioned before, Paleo is not a diet. A diet has limits, but the Paleo way of thinking can be adapted to everything related to food, recipes, baking and cooking that your mind desires. Be as creative with it as you like, but just respect the Paleo rules that you can refer back to in the beginning of this book.

We chose to demonstrate Paleo with dessert recipes so that you do understand this powerful lifestyle that you can create for yourself. Usually, dessert recipes are associated by society with guilt and shame, but at the same time with pleasure. To show you the power of Paleo we chose the toughest type of food that is desserts in order to show you how paleo can even be applied to sugar and guilt loaded desserts.

As you got started reading the book, you probably thought guilt free desserts no way and it looked impossible and suspicious to you to turn desirable desserts that are associated with guilt into something guilt free.

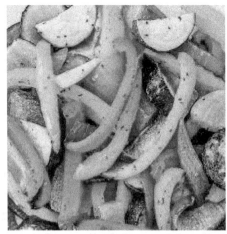

This book is going to enables you to figure out the problem how to turn any desired food type like desserts into a pleasure that is guilt free because it respects the rules of the Paleo lifestyle.

Once you have figured out this problem you are in the zone, at least mentally, so we congratulate you on reading through the book and getting the knowledge that you need in order to make this lifestyle change a successful one.

Make sure to go to the next step and that is taking action. Make sure to have a clear goal in mind and get started with one or two recipes and explore more from there.

Now you have learned that Paleo is not something like a diet that comes with limits, but you have been able to see with your very own eyes how even desserts that we desire and love eating but that we have been conditioned not to eat so much because they are bad for us can be turned into a an exciting new experience that is far away from feeling guilty about something like desserts.

We encourage you to explore this lifestyle further on your own and have fun to find out many other guilt free Paleo recipe applications for yourself. This knowledge empowers you to explore new levels and dimensions of eating that you have never thought possible before.

Do not let anybody tell you that this is not the way to go. Do not become discouraged if little things do not turn out right once in a while. Keep trying until you reach your goal. Once you are able to see it and apply it to your daily meal plan, you will never want to go back to your past eating habits.

Once you are able to apply Paleo to all your food choices, you will feel the magical power of Paleo and that is when you are living the Paleo Lifestyle!

CPSIA information can be obtained
at www.ICGtesting.com
Printed in the USA
BVHW011109190321
602997BV00009B/380